THE COMPLETE IDIOT'S GUIDE® TO

Working Out with a Partner

Illustrated

by Aimee Labrecque and Ted Vickey

ALPHA

A member of Penguin Group (USA) Inc.

International Standard Book Number: 1-59257-244-8
Library of Congress Catalog Card Number: 2004106742

06   05   04   8   7   6   5   4   3   2   1

Interpretation of the printing code: The rightmost number of the first series of numbers is the year of the book's printing; the rightmost number of the second series of numbers is the number of the book's printing. For example, a printing code of 04-1 shows that the first printing occurred in 2004.

Printed in the United States of America

Note: This publication contains the opinions and ideas of its authors. It is intended to provide helpful and informative material on the subject matter covered. It is sold with the understanding that the authors and publisher are not engaged in rendering professional services in the book. If the reader requires personal assistance or advice, a competent professional should be consulted.

The authors and publisher specifically disclaim any responsibility for any liability, loss, or risk, personal or otherwise, which is incurred as a consequence, directly or indirectly, of the use and application of any of the contents of this book.

Most Alpha books are available at special quantity discounts for bulk purchases for sales promotions, premiums, fund-raising, or educational use. Special books, or book excerpts, can also be created to fit specific needs.

For details, write: Special Markets, Alpha Books, 375 Hudson Street, New York, NY 10014.

Publisher: *Marie Butler-Knight*
Product Manager: *Phil Kitchel*
Senior Managing Editor: *Jennifer Chisholm*
Senior Acquisitions Editor: *Mike Sanders*
Development Editor: *Michael Thomas*
Production Editor: *Megan Douglass*
Copy Editor: *Jeff Rose*
Illustrator: *Richard King*
Cover/Book Designer: *Trina Wurst*
Indexer: *Heather McNeil*
Layout/Proofreading: *Becky Harmon*

Contents at a Glance

Contents

Foreword

For many individuals, starting an exercise program can be a daunting task. Even if they do get started, they inevitably have days when they simply don't feel like exercising. Human nature being what it is, that first missed workout often makes it easier for a person to miss the next workout and eventually stop exercising altogether. As such, one of the key issues with regard to working out is how can individuals stay motivated to stick with their exercise routines?

Available evidence (research based and anecdotal) suggests that individuals are far less likely to miss their scheduled workouts if it means letting another person down. It has been my personal and professional experience that exercising with a partner not only enhances exercise adherence, it also offers many additional benefits including heightened motivation, improved safety, increased social interaction, and healthy competition.

In *The Complete Idiot's Guide to Working Out with a Partner Illustrated*, you'll find a wide variety of useful tips on how to effectively take advantage of exercising with a partner. This book offers individuals of all ages and fitness levels a user-friendly guide on developing overall fitness. It provides solid, easy-to-understand information on a wide variety of fitness activities that can be safely and effectively performed with a partner (for example, aerobic exercise, strength training, stretching, yoga, and Pilates).

The Complete Idiot's Guide to Working Out with a Partner Illustrated was written to help you—whether you're just starting to work out or want to modify or enhance your current training program. I found the information dealing with selecting the "right" partner and how to be a good exercise partner to be particularly helpful. The authors also do an outstanding job of providing practical tips and advice on how to make exercising with a partner a win-win proposition.

Clearly written and well illustrated, this book is must reading for anyone interested in protecting their most valuable asset—their health. The authors of *The Complete Idiot's Guide to Working Out with a Partner Illustrated* have provided a straightforward road map to help you and your exercise partner safely experience the joys and innumerable benefits of a physically active lifestyle. This book will help you learn strategies to combat exercise boredom and to keep you going when you are tempted to remain on the couch. I hope you enjoy it as much as I did.

Cedric X. Bryant, Ph.D., FACSM
Chief Exercise Physiologist and Vice President of Educational Services
American Council on Exercise
San Diego, CA

Introduction

Welcome aboard your fitness partner journey. Whether this is the first fitness book you've ever purchased, or whether it's one of many, we certainly hope it will be the only one you'll need (until we write a second edition, of course!). You see, we believe so strongly in the concept of fitness partners as a way to achieve fitness success that we're sure after you breeze through the pages of this book, you'll never need to purchase another workout book again. How can we be so sure?

The reason is simply stated by the Double Mint twins. You remember those commercials from the 1980s for stick gum, right? They always featured two identical twins chewing gum who always ended the commercial by saying, "Double your pleasure, double your fun." Little did those twins know it, but they were laying the foundation for this very book. They were exercising together and having fun and that's what this book is all about. Okay, so maybe chewing gum isn't exactly exercise, but it does work your muscles of mastication, so we think that counts! The point is that if you want to stick to an exercise plan, you have to have fun while doing it. And if you want to have fun while doing it, you can't do it alone.

What You'll Find in This Book

This book is divided into four parts. **Part 1, "It Takes Two,"** is all about finding the right partner and starting your exercise plan. Readers will learn what to look for in a partner to guarantee fitness success and the types of personality conflicts to avoid. "It Takes Two" also takes a closer look at the ways you can measure your fitness success in addition to just the numbers on the bathroom scale.

Part 2, "Gonna Make You Sweat," contains everything you need to know about beginning a cardiovascular exercise program. In this part we dive deep into aerobic activity and the different kinds of workouts that you and your partner can do together. You'll learn to measure how hard you are working and when to increase the intensity of your workouts. This part also includes sample workouts to get you started.

Part 3, "Muscle Madness," is about uncovering the mysteries of strength training. You'll learn how to organize your workout session to get the most out of your muscles. You'll also learn about the importance of rest and recovery to building long, lean muscles. In this part you will also be instructed about the equipment that you can purchase to keep your workouts challenging and effective.

Part 4, "Stretch Your Limits," covers the often forgotten component of exercise—flexibility. This part not only discusses the importance of stretching, but highlights the many different types of stretching programs, including yoga and Pilates. Partners will learn how to safely stretch each other to avoid injury and increase their muscle potential.

The *Work It Out* chapters are the actual exercise chapters where we illustrate the exercises you'll be doing with your partner. These chapters also include all of the pictures that you no doubt have already looked at, because who buys a book without looking at the pictures first?

In addition to the fancy pictures, we think you'll enjoy this book because it takes a lighthearted approach to a subject that can be complex and sometimes emotional for some readers. The key is to put down your defenses and any preconceived notions you may have about exercise. When you do this, you will be able to open yourself up to a new kind of fitness journey, one where we're sure you'll find success.

Don't Miss This

We've added some tidbits of information throughout the book. These little sidebars are there to provide insight, clarity, and sometimes they are just stuck in there to make you laugh. In any case, here's what you should look for:

Fit Facts

Hints about health or fitness that may help make your life and your workouts a little easier.

Training Notes

Definitions of terms that are used throughout the text. These terms can also be found in the glossary at the back of the book.

Workout Worries

Warnings that alert you to possible dangers or potential for injury. Read these and you'll steer clear of the injury corner.

Don't Sweat It

Notes that provide additional information about a topic discussed in the text.

Acknowledgments

This book would not have been possible without the support of so many people.

Aimee would like to thank her parents, Terene and Dave, who have proven to be the truest partners, in fitness and life, and an inspiration to her every day. She would also like to thank her siblings, Keri, Kevin, Nicole, and George, for proving that parenting is the hardest workout of them all.

Ted would like to thank his parents, Fred and Nancy, for their commitment to the family values and as role models (Mom recently has lost 40 pounds—way to go, Mom); his siblings for their willingness to live with such a wonderful older brother (Colleen, Tim, Buzz, Maggie, and Katie); and all the members of Team FitWell, CHS, our clients, and our thousands of client members who make each day a joy to live.

To the people whose brilliance contributed in some way to the work in this book: RJ Ross, Ari Gonzales, Lauren Labrecque, Mike Masella, Amanda Cristoe, Eric Stanley, Dave Schwalbe, Brian Reisenberg, and Andrew Slye.

Special thanks to John Szpara, our photographer, who labored tirelessly to make all of our models look great in these pictures.

Please contact us:

fitnesspartners@fitwellinc.com

Trademarks

All terms mentioned in this book that are known to be or are suspected of being trademarks or service marks have been appropriately capitalized. Alpha Books and Penguin Group (USA) Inc. cannot attest to the accuracy of this information. Use of a term in this book should not be regarded as affecting the validity of any trademark or service mark.

In This Part

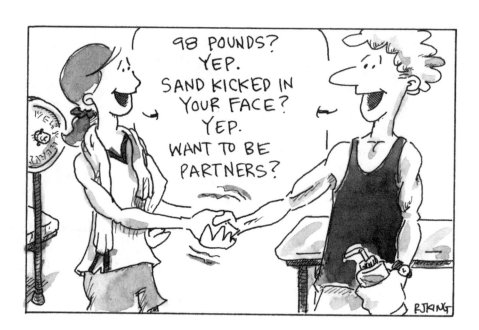

Part 1

It Takes Two

Coming together is a beginning. Keeping together is progress.
Working together is success.

—Henry Ford

It would be easy to start another exercise program by yourself. You could gear up for big weight loss success, vowing to finally get that perfect body you always knew was possible. You could change your diet, start to exercise, and motivate yourself to become "the new you."

Then somewhere down the line, after a few lost pounds and clothing sizes, you'd start to fall off the wagon. One missed workout here, one extra donut there. Before you know it, the pounds and the clothing sizes are back and you have disappointed yourself once again.

But you're through with disappointment and fitness failures! You are ready to embark on a more rewarding fitness journey. You are ready to find a fitness partner.

This partner is going to be your cheerleader, personal trainer, and motivational speaker. This partner is going to pick you up when you're down and drag you out of bed before you can hit the snooze button. This partnership is the ticket to your fitness success.

In This Chapter

- ◆ The benefits of having an exercise partner
- ◆ Why exercising with a partner is better than exercising alone
- ◆ What you can expect from your exercise partnership
- ◆ How your fitness partnership can guarantee fitness success

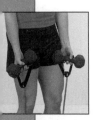
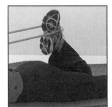
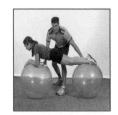
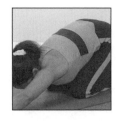
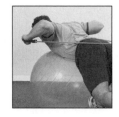
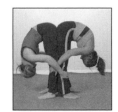

Chapter 1

Two's Company

You might be asking yourself why you bought this book in the first place. After all, you already know you want to exercise and you know you don't want to do it alone. It should be that simple. Find a partner and start working out, right?

But why do you need a partner? What can you accomplish with a partner that you wouldn't be able to on your own? What are the benefits of having someone by your side as you begin your fitness journey?

This chapter will help you answer many of those questions. In this chapter, you will learn why you might need a partner and how that partnership will affect your exercise success. We'll point out some "partner perks" that you may not have even thought about and how these little bonuses will help ensure a happy outcome at the gym.

Who Needs a Partner?

We're going to go out on a limb and assume that you've already considered the reasons why you might need an exercise partner. Maybe you've reflected upon your previous attempts at starting an exercise program and found that you lacked the support and encouragement you needed to succeed. Possibly you have determined that you fall into that category of people who have more success when they pair up with someone to achieve a goal. Or maybe you know you'll just have more fun if you bring your sidekick to your workouts so you can suffer through the sweat together.

Whatever the reason, needing a partner should not be viewed as a weakness or short-coming. It's actually a great thing. It means you are a team player and you welcome other people to share your challenges. There are plenty of people out there who work better alone. This does not make them stronger or more capable than you. It just makes them, well, alone. But realizing that your fitness efforts will be complimented by adding a partner is a great thing. We're proud of you for taking this first step.

Workout Worries

If you have made several attempts at adopting an exercise program by your-self and failed, chances are that you don't have the right amount of support and motivation to continue. Don't make the same mistake again. Try out a fitness partner for six weeks. This is long enough to start to develop a habit. We guarantee you'll be hooked!

Now if you are not exactly certain that a partner is what you need, ask yourself these questions:

- Do you often get bored while exercising?
- Do you spend more time at the gym conversing with others than working out?
- Are you stuck in a workout rut and looking for something or someone to take you to the next level?
- Are you too intimidated to start exercising at a fitness center or health club?
- Do you have great fitness goals but no idea how to achieve them?
- Do you often set your health and fitness goals too high and get discouraged when you don't achieve them?

If you can agree with any of these statements, then you need an exercise partner. Everyone can benefit from the support of a fitness partner. You don't need to be out of shape, in great shape, a loner, or a party animal. Fitness partners are for everyone. Need more reasons why?

Cheap Man's Personal Training

Now we're calling you cheap. How do you like that?

Maybe you have already considered hiring a personal trainer to help you in your quest to become fit. If so, then you've probably already realized that this is going to cost you a couple of hard-earned bucks. Experienced trainers don't often come cheap, nor should they. Their services are valuable and should not be under-estimated. However, if you are not yet willing to make that kind of investment, your fitness partner is the perfect replacement. This is the beauty of a fitness partner—all the benefits of a personal trainer, but none of the cash!

Similar to a personal trainer, your fitness partner will be able to …

- motivate you on the days you don't feel like exercising.
- help you define and achieve your exercise goals.
- assist you in executing exercises safely and properly.
- encourage you to push beyond your limits.
- help you monitor your progress and celebrate successes along the way.
- provide emotional support and a listening ear.

Keeping in mind that your fitness partner cannot replace the value of a certified personal trainer, they sure can make a great substitute if you are not ready to fork over the money to hire a trainer of your own.

The Security Blanket

When you think of your local health club, do you conjure up images of twenty-somethings in tank tops exposing pockets of muscle you didn't know existed except on the medical posters in doctor's offices? Do you embrace the fitness center subculture of spandex and sports bras with about as much enthusiasm as a root canal? Have you uttered these statements: "I need to lose weight before I start going to the gym." Or "Everyone at the gym is in good shape."

While most fitness centers try to cater to the needs of all fitness levels, it is often the case that most of the participants already seem to be in great shape. This can be intimidating if you are the newcomer. Your good intentions of starting an exercise program can easily be thwarted when you walk in to the gym on your first day to find a sea of fit people in tight clothing. While this may be more of an illusion than actual truth, it is true that a fitness center and its participants can be intimidating when you are in less than perfect shape.

If you can relate to any of these feelings, you may be suffering from what we like to call "gym jitters." Don't worry, gym jitters are ugly, but curable. You just need the right dose of support and encouragement from none other than your wonderful fitness partner. Safety in numbers is what we call it. If you and your partner can challenge the fitness center stigma together, chances are you can overcome the intimidation factor and become regular gym-goers. Remember, your fitness partner is your best ally when it comes to expanding your comfort zone. Don't let fears stand in the way of your goals. Just throw on your fitness partner safety blanket and jump in!

Workout Worries

Gym jitters don't have to stand in your way of getting the most from your fitness program. Don't forget, most of the fit people you see in gyms today were once in your shoes. They were intimidated and afraid to participate, and now they are at the front of the class. Don't hold back. Jump into the gym scene with your fitness partner!

Double Your Pleasure, Double Your Fun!

We realize that you are still getting used to the idea that fitness just might be fun, so you can read this section with a little bit of caution if you must.

The problem with exercise is that it's work. And it's hard work, at that. Most people don't exactly embrace hard physical labor. Rather, they find a million excuses to avoid it. What most people forget is that although most instances that require hard physical labor don't come with the promise of a "good time" attached to it, they usually result in feelings of success and satisfaction. Think childbirth or running a marathon. The challenge with strenuous activity is to find the "good time" before you get to the end, and then you just might be likely to repeat the activity again and again.

Enter the multifaceted fitness partner! Personal trainer, security blanket, and now, stand-up comedian! While your partner may not be a barrel of laughs all the time, we think you two will be able to make a "good time" out of your fitness adventure. You just need to get creative. Here are some reasons why fitness with a partner is more fun than fitness alone:

◆ **It Takes Two to Tango.** That's right. You and your partner can take a dance class. The two of you two-stepping—now that sounds like fun!

- **The Team Effort.** Get involved in a sport like tennis that requires two people. You'll be getting your workout and enjoying the competition.

- **Chatting It Up.** A great time to catch up and share stories is during your workouts. It's like telling stories over dinner, except you're burning calories instead of consuming them!

- **Be an Athletic Supporter.** Sometimes what you need in life is a cheerleader, someone to root you on through life's challenges. Any tough obstacle can be made more fun with a little support. You can count on your fitness partner to be your biggest fan.

- **Become a Dynamic Duo.** You'll be able to leap tall buildings in a single bound! Wonder Twin Powers, activate! While you may not reach superhero proportions, don't be surprised if you and your partner start getting recognized around the gym as the "Dynamic Duo." Notoriety is not a bad thing.

If you are not sold yet, then just trust us. Fitness is more fun if you have a sidekick. Hey, if it works for the Double Mint twins, why not you?

Don't Sweat It

"The world is your playground. Why aren't you playing?"

—Ellie Katz

Commit to Get Fit

Any good personal relationship starts with goals. And in order to achieve those goals, there needs to be a solid commitment on the part of both individuals. The commitment phase of a relationship defines each party's dedication to the goals. Without that commitment, the partnership goals may become undermined by individual goals, which inevitably leads toward breakdown and breakup. Whew! How's that for psychobabble?

What we're trying to point out here is that by having a partner, you are making a commitment with someone to set goals and to achieve those goals. It's the greatest thing about a fitness partnership—the commitment.

Now maybe you're one of those commitment-phobic types and right now are thinking you're not so sure about taking that step into a relationship with a fitness partner. You realize that by entering into this relationship, you're accepting the responsibility of helping another person achieve their goals. This, to you, might be a huge commitment. Yikes! There's that word again!

Fear not! We are here to talk you out of commitment phobia and into a very healthy relationship. You see, committing to get fit with someone is not just about making a promise to exercise for an hour a day, three days per week together. It's really about embracing the challenge of changing your lifestyle in a positive way to better not only yourself, but someone else, too. At the risk of sounding overly dramatic, this is a beautiful thing!

The trick to embracing your fitness commitment is to have a complete understanding of the relationship expectations. For this, you and your partner should sit down and define your level of commitment to each other. In relationship terms, try to think of this as the prenuptial agreement without the money issues!

As a fitness partner you are committing to …

- establish and stick to a workout schedule with your partner.

- motivate your partner through each workout session.

- constructively evaluate your partner's progress and make suggestions for improvement.
- support your partner when they hit a bump in the road.
- provide positive feedback when your partner makes great strides.
- make every workout session enjoyable and fun!

Fit Facts

To avoid fitness commitment phobia, define the parameters of your relationship with your partner. If you know exactly what is expected of you, then what is there to fear? When defining your relationship, specifically address:

- How often you will exercise together
- Where your workouts will take place
- How you will support and encourage each other
- Any special needs each partner may have
- Any other obligations that will interfere with your fitness commitment

So take that first step and commit to get fit!

The Least You Need to Know

- If you've had several failed attempts at maintaining an exercise program, it's time to get a partner.
- The fitness partnership should include a commitment to support, encourage, and motivate each other during the relationship.
- Having a fitness partner can be just like having a personal trainer, only cheaper.
- Having a fitness partner brings fun into the fitness game.

In This Chapter

- ◆ Are you "fit" to be a fitness partner?

- ◆ The importance of sampling potential workout partners

- ◆ When spouses and friends make great partners— and when they don't

- ◆ How to avoid overcommitment

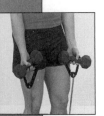
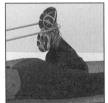
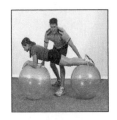
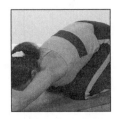
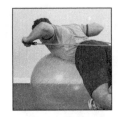
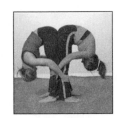

Chapter 2

Teaming Up

Since committing to begin your exercise program, you've probably purchased some spiffy new workout gear to get you started. Possibly it was some new sneakers or the latest moisture-wicking clothing for your upcoming sweat sessions. No doubt you shopped around, tried on several items and chose the ones that were comfortable and fit you best. Maybe you considered style and looks for your new sneakers and maybe all you cared about was that you didn't end up with a blister on your big toe! But in all of your shopping outings, did you ever stop to think how you would "shop" for your exercise partner?

We're here to tell you that finding an exercise partner is a lot like finding that comfortable pair of sneakers. In this chapter, we'll guide you through the process of selecting the right workout partner to meet not only your fitness needs, but your emotional needs as well. We'll give you tips on where to find potential partners and how to pick the weeds out of a bunch of roses. Now let's head to the dressing room and try out some new partners!

First: Choose You!

Congratulations! You have just been promoted to a new position in life. Your new title is Fitness Partner Extraordinaire and your job description is quite lengthy. You may want to get out a pen. This new position requires you to be a motivator, counselor, cheerleader, therapist, doctor, consultant, and most important, a friend. This is your mission should you choose to accept it.

Wait a minute, wait a minute, wait a minute! Are you confused? After all, you thought you bought this book so we would help you find all those qualities in a partner for you. You didn't think you were going to get off easy, did you? On the contrary, my friend. This fitness partnership is a two-way street and you first need to make sure you're driving on the right side of the road. Are you ready for this? Are you prepared to be all those things we just mentioned and more to your workout buddy? We hope so, because that's what it takes to be involved in a successful fitness relationship. Sweat and soreness is only one part of the battle. The other lies in your ability to keep your partner motivated and streamlined for success inside and outside of the gym. So what do you say? Can you do it? Yes, you can!

Workout Worries

The Fitness Partnership is not just about exercising with your buddy. It is a relationship just like any other and requires support, encouragement, and communication to succeed.

Your Needs and Expectations

Okay, now that you've chosen your Mission Possible, it's time get down to business. Let's start by defining your needs and expectations for your upcoming partnership. This can be a simple process of outlining some basic guidelines to help narrow your search when you take to the streets to find your fitness soul mate. Consider some of the following questions during your defining moment:

◆ **What are my exercise goals?** If your goal is to lose ten pounds for your high school reunion and your partner needs to lose fifty pounds for health reasons, this may not be the best union. You and your partner's goals do not need to be identical, but they should be similar to achieve success.

◆ **Am I a morning exerciser or evening exerciser?** If your partner rises with the sun and you don't start feeling your oats until the sun goes down, you may want to ditch the rooster for a night owl. Well-meaning partners can adapt to each other's schedules, but old habits are hard to break. Look for someone whose clock is ticking at the same pace as yours.

◆ **Does sex matter?** Get your mind out of the gutter. We're talking about gender! Sometimes females prefer female partners and males prefer male partners. Keep in mind that this exercise process can bring about a lot of physical and emotional changes, all of which can be very personal. Consider who you would feel most comfortable sharing those feelings with.

◆ **What are my motivational needs?** Do you need a gentle push or a swift kick in the pants? Look for someone who can match your needs and bring out your best performance. If you need a drill sergeant, choosing your church mouse neighbor may not suit. You want someone who will get you to the gym on the days you don't want to go and push you past every plateau along the way.

Fit Facts

If you're unsure of whether you are a morning or evening exerciser, try this: Set your alarm one hour earlier every morning for one week. Then get up and do some light exercise. If you can't wait for the week to end so you can go back to sleeping later, you probably aren't a morning exerciser!

This second step in the partner selection process (the first one was choosing yourself, in case you forgot) is a critical one. Knowing what your needs are will help to weed out potential partners who don't fit your mold. Remember: While this fitness partnership is a 50/50 relationship, your needs are 100 percent important to you.

You Who?

Now that you've determined what your needs in this workout relationship will be, it's time to find a potential mate. Maybe you have a few individuals in mind who you would consider teaming up with—a co-worker who works the same long hours as you, a neighbor who you see walking every morning when you fetch your paper, or your sister who's desperately trying to squeeze into her high school prom dress (which just happens to be the same dress you wore!). If you can think of a short list of people, great! You are ahead of the game and well on your way to finding the perfect partner.

However let's assume for the moment that no one in your life is begging to join your exercise crusade. Or should we assume there is no one in your life you would like to spend one hour per day, three to four days per week getting to know intimately as you share each other's sweat and glory? In either case, you are stuck without a prospective partner and we need to help you out. Here are a few suggestions for soliciting that special someone:

◆ **Post a flyer at your fitness facility.** Many fitness centers have a member bulletin board for exactly this purpose. If there is no such space for member use, consider using word of mouth. Let other members know that you are looking for a workout buddy. You are your best advertisement. Show your dedication and commitment around the gym, and like-minded individuals will be drawn to you.

Fit Facts

If you are posting your flyer in a familiar place like your fitness facility, consider adding your picture. People are more likely to respond to your inquiry if they recognize your face from around the gym.

◆ **Network in other circles.** Maybe the president of your garden club has been looking to start an exercise program. After all, gardening is good exercise, so you're already off to a good start! Let everyone you come in contact with know you are looking for an exercise partner. You might find your perfect partner in the strangest of places. Think grocery store checkout line.

◆ **Check online resources.** There are several websites dedicated to pairing up fitness partners including www.usatrainingpartners.com. These sites can be great tools for finding people in your area interested in teaming up. As with any website, check the credentials before submitting personal information.

◆ **Post a flyer on neighborhood or community bulletin boards.** Most grocery stores these days have community boards where local vendors and service providers advertise. Consider posting your flyer in one of these places. Who knows, you might find an exercise partner and a babysitter in the same day!

Swing That Partner

The recruiting phase is over. You are sizing up your potential candidates and your decision is a difficult one. Well then, it's time to take your top recruits for a swing around the square. This is a sort of test drive with you in the driver and passenger seats. The purpose of the sample workout is to see how you and your potential partner will get along during an exercise session. This is matchmaking at its best, so put your best foot forward! (That's fitness humor for you newbies!) This union may not be as significant as finding your potential lifelong mate, but it's been our experience that fitness partnerships often last longer than most romantic relationships, so don't make this decision lightly.

In order to get the most out of the test drive, be prepared to answer these questions along the way:

◆ **Are our fitness levels similar?** If you are struggling to keep up with your partner, consider how this may hinder your progress. While every train needs a caboose, you don't always want to be the one bringing up the rear.

◆ **Do we have similar interests and values?** This may not seem so important at the start, but just wait until you are on a forty-minute powerwalk with nothing to talk about. Sharing interests can lead to hours of endless conversation which will make your workouts much more enjoyable.

◆ **Which habits will eventually annoy me?** Okay, we're not asking you to pick apart your partner and look for flaws. However we're sure you know what we're talking about here. Simple things like talking too much or breathing too loudly can really drive you nuts after an hour in the gym. Chances are if you found it slightly irritating in a single workout session, it will make your skin crawl after several months.

◆ **Can I communicate with this person?** We all know that good communication is the key to any successful relationship, and fitness partnering is no exception. During your sample session, look for signs of communication pitfalls. Can you be totally honest with this person? Are you intimidated by this person? Are you afraid to share your opinions with this person? All of these barriers will lead to major obstacles as your relationship continues.

◆ **Does this person challenge me to push my limits?** There is a term in exercise physiology called the *overload principle*. In short, it requires the exerciser to push beyond his or her previous limits in order to achieve progress. It is absolutely essential that your fitness partner help you push past the limits you set in your previous workout if you want to increase your fitness potential.

Training Notes

The **overload principle** is the necessity to push the body beyond its previous limit in order to achieve progress. It's lifting more weight the next day than you did the day before or adding one more city block to your powerwalk as your fitness improves.

Love and Fitness: The Kiss of Death?

It was bound to cross your mind: Your significant other as your workout partner. Is this a match made in heaven or does the mere thought of exercising with him or her make your heart rate climb? You've come this far, you are committed to your health and fitness goals. Is your partner the right person to work out with? Easy question, tough answers. Before you decide to

make your significant other your workout partner, consider The Good, The Bad, and The
Ugly:

◆ **The Good**—You've talked about wanting
to spend more time with each other and
your days are already hectic. Why not kill
two birds with one stone? (P.S.—We
don't condone killing or stoning anything.) Share a walk in the park, a round
of golf, or a spin on the bike, and spend
time with each other.

◆ **The Bad**—Your decision to begin an
exercise program is propelled by your
desire to get away from your partner or
spouse and work off the stress of the relationship. Now we're fitness professionals,
not marriage counselors, but we're going
to go out on a limb and say that person
would make a poor fitness partner. Truth
be told, we don't think your workout, let
alone your relationship, will succeed.

◆ **The Ugly**—You were going to choose
your significant other as your workout
partner, but then you met this very cute
gym member at your local health club.
Turns out you have more in common with
this Mr. Buff Bod than with your current
mate. So in an effort to maximize your
relationship potential inside and outside
of the gym, you're trading in your old
mate for the upgraded version. Ouch!

For the sake of this discussion, let's assume
The Good holds true. Will this utopian view
of love and fitness really withstand the sweat
and gruel? In most cases, we're going to say
yes! Romantic partners can make great fitness
buddies. Here are some terrific reasons to
choose your mate as your fitness date:

◆ **Your health is important to both of
you.** Who is more qualified (besides your
doctor) to care about your health and
wellness than your spouse or significant

other? We have had countless couples
who were concerned about each other's
health come to us for guidance and training. They made a commitment to each
other to get fit and planned to take the
necessary steps together.

◆ **Your schedules will likely be similar.**
In most cases, you share similar routines
with your spouse or significant other.
Finding the time to exercise together may
not be as much of a challenge as finding
the time with a friend or acquaintance. Or
at the worst, it will require minimal man-
euvering of schedules to make it happen.

◆ **You can provide daily encouragement/
reminders to each other.** While some
might consider it nagging to have that
angel sitting on your shoulder when you
pass by the fast food restaurant, others
find it helpful to have a continual reminder
of their fitness commitment. It has been
proven that family support is one of the
greatest indicators of weight loss success.

◆ **Exercise is an aphrodisiac.** Need we say
more? It's a little-known fact that exercise
causes an increase in the level of *endorphins*
in your body. These hormones are also
found in elevated levels during times of
sexual arousal. If you don't believe that
scientific hub-bub, believe this: Exercise
can increase your self-esteem, leaving you
feeling great about yourself and your body.
This can mean great things for your romantic relationships. We'll leave it at that.

Training Notes

Endorphins are hormones released
into the bloodstream during exercise. These
hormones are related to mood elevation
and feelings of euphoria and are the same
substances released into the bloodstream
during sexual arousal.

After that last item, we're sure you're ready to run off and enlist your lover in your exercise adventure. However we wouldn't be doing our job if we didn't share with you the flip side of the coin:

◆ **Family Obligations**—This is where things can get tricky, especially if there are children involved. You may find it difficult to keep your workout commitments to each other between soccer practice, piano lessons, and Boy Scout meetings. Be realistic. If you and your partner have difficulty finding time to share a dinner or movie alone, chances are that scheduling an hour or two at the gym is out of the question.

◆ **Jealousy Issues**—In most instances, we like to think that partners will always be supportive of each other's health and wellness goals. After all, who doesn't want their partner looking and feeling great? (Refer to the aforementioned aphrodisiac commentary if you've forgotten!) However, in rare cases, the fitness success of one partner can lead to jealousy on the part of the other. This is due in part to feelings of insecurity that extend far beyond weight loss or weight gain. Whatever the cause, if your partner is prone to jealousy, you may not get the support you're looking for when trying to reach your fitness goals.

Workout Worries

If you choose to work out with your partner or close friend, consider the triggers and traps that will bar you from meeting your fitness goals. For instance, will your intimate relationship make it easier to be unmotivated (and head out for ice cream) than stick to your original exercise plan?

Two's Company, Three's a Crowd

It might have worked for Jack, Janet, and Chrissy in that '70s sitcom, *Three's Company*, but in most cases, three is definitely a crowd. We are certainly not discouraging you from exercising in groups. As a matter of fact, we highly encourage it in future chapters, so keep reading. Our word of caution about large groups of exercise buddies is more about simplicity and practicality. Doesn't it always seem that things get done faster, more effectively, and most successfully when fewer people are involved in the equation? More does not always mean merrier. The more people you invite in to your group, the greater the chances of having your exercise plans sidelined. Here's why:

◆ **Too many schedules to work around.** Coordinating the schedules of several people is a lot like trying to balance the national budget. Just when you think you have all the numbers in place, inevitably something will arise to throw all of your equations off. If you're lucky enough to find a time when everyone can exercise together, your plans will no doubt be thwarted by family obligations, work commitments, or personal emergencies. While a certain amount of flexibility is necessary to a successful fitness partnership, bending to the will of several participants will kill your exercise momentum quickly.

◆ **Too much chatter.** Yeah, yeah. We know. Just a few short pages ago we were encouraging you to find a partner you could talk to. Now we're telling you to shut up. What gives, you ask? It's just that too much talking can get in the way of productive exercise. It's human nature for people who share a common interest to talk. That's probably what brought you together in the first place. You started talking about a finding a fitness partner and then boom! You found five. Kudos for your recruiting abilities, but at some point talk needs to become action. Unfortunately, the more people you have in the group, the greater the likelihood that water cooler gossip will overrun your fitness initiatives. So here's a good rule of thumb: If your mouth is moving, the rest of you better be moving as well.

◆ **Too much commitment.** When we started this chapter, we told you that the fitness partnership involved being a motivator, counselor, cheerleader, therapist, doctor, consultant, and most important, a friend. Well, there is such a thing as being too many things to too many people. And as the exercise routine progresses and more physical and emotional changes come into play, you may find yourself overextended if you are committed to too many partners. The last thing you want to do is spend all of your energy keeping everyone else happy. You probably have enough of that going on in your life already.

It's important to note that we do not discourage exercising in groups. The group atmosphere provides a great sense of camaraderie for most participants. We simply caution against committing yourself to too many people at one time. Before you know it, you will be woven into a tangled web of scheduling, canceling, rescheduling, and ultimately missing your precious workouts.

Spot the Spotter

When we set out to write this book, we made the assumption that you were looking for a human fitness partner. However we would be remiss if we did not acknowledge the effectiveness of your pet as your fitness partner. After all, what kind of dog doesn't like a run in the park after being cooped up all day? The lazy kind, we suppose. In any case, we felt it necessary to mention how great Spot can be when your human fitness partner is unavailable or has to cancel.

◆ **Spot never cancels on you.** Have you ever had your dog tell you he couldn't make his afternoon walk with you due to work commitments? (Work with us here. Assume your dog could talk to you for this case. Note: If your dog does talk to you, seek professional counseling immediately.)

◆ **Spot is always happy to exercise.** You never have to convince Spot to play fetch. He's ready to go when you are.

◆ **Spot does not complain.** Unlike your human fitness partner who may occasionally grumble as you wake her up for your 6 A.M. powerwalk, Spot will always greet you with his happy bark.

◆ **Spot always agrees with you.** Should we walk or run? You'll always get your way with Spot by your side.

So doggone it, in a pinch, pick Spot!

The Least You Need to Know

◆ A fitness partnership is not just a commitment to exercise. It's a relationship that involves support, encouragement, and communication.

◆ Knowing your own emotional and fitness needs will help you find a compatible partner.

◆ Sometimes spouses and significant others make great exercise partners. Sometimes they just don't.

◆ It is possible to overcommit yourself to too many people, so avoid getting involved with multiple partners.

In This Chapter

- What you should know before starting a workout program with your partner

- The importance of baseline measurements for charting your fitness program success

- How to set goals with your partner that you can actually accomplish

- Tools for evaluating the success of your fitness partnership

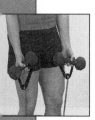
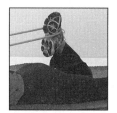
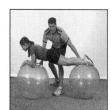
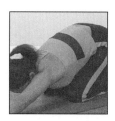
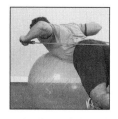
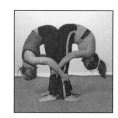

Chapter 3

The Rules of Engagement

Now that you've found the perfect fitness partner, it's time to get down to business. How often are you going to exercise together? What are your fitness goals and what are your partner's? Are you going to write a fitness contract?

Hey, we're not kidding about the contract. Your health is serious business. We want to make sure you get exactly what you deserve out of this fitness partnership. Anything less and you will have another unsuccessful attempt at getting in shape and adopting a healthier lifestyle. We don't want to be responsible for that failure, so this chapter is full of tips and information to make sure that your new partnership is a success.

What's Your Baseline?

We're going to ask you a tough question: What kind of shape are you in right now? Chances are, if we could ask you this question in person, we wouldn't get an honest answer anyway. That's not to say that you would lie to us, but maybe you just don't know what kind of shape you are in. You may think that this information is not important. After all, you already know you want to "get in shape" or "lose some weight," so what does it matter what your fitness abilities are right now?

Actually, it matters very much. Having a good idea of your current fitness level will help you measure how much you improve during your fitness program. Many people shy away from taking measurements when they start working out because they don't want to know how out of shape they are. But trust us. Knowing these baseline numbers will help you chart your progress, stay motivated by your success, and set goals to make improvements. The best advice we can give is to take the measurements, record them somewhere, and then forget about them. Don't obsess about the numbers. They don't mean anything right now anyway.

Workout Worries

Don't get too concerned about what your baseline measurements say about your current fitness level. These numbers only become important after you have been exercising regularly and are seeing results. Then you can retake your measurements and see how far you've come. A show of improvement will keep you motivated to continue on your fitness journey.

So if we've sold you on the idea of getting some numbers on paper, what measurements should you take?

Body Weight

One of the most commonly used methods of tracking fitness is body weight. However just because it's the most common does not mean that it's the best. Your body weight can change throughout the day, so depending on when, where, and how you weigh yourself, your weight will vary. For the average American, stepping on the bathroom scale is the easiest way to measure their fitness.

Fit Facts

Avoid weighing yourself too often. Most fitness professionals recommend weighing yourself once per week. Because your weight can fluctuate throughout the day, be sure to weigh yourself at the same time, on the same scale, wearing the same amount of clothing. This will give you the most accurate recording each time.

The following chart is the most widely used height and weight chart, first established by Metropolitan Life Insurance Company in 1943 and then updated in 1983. To see how you fit in, compare your weight (in pounds) with the range for the same height and build. The charts assume three pounds for clothing, so if you are weighing yourself without clothes, subtract three pounds from the chart. Only use this chart for comparison purposes. We don't really recommend height and weight charts for determining your overall fitness level.

Height and Weight Table For Women

Height	Small Frame	Medium Frame	Large Frame
4' 10"	102-111	109-121	181-131
4' 11"	103-113	111-123	120-134
5' 0"	104-115	113-126	122-137
5' 1"	106-118	115-129	125-140
5' 2"	108-121	118-132	128-143
5' 3"	111-124	121-135	131-147
5' 4"	114-127	124-138	134-151
5' 5"	117-130	127-141	137-155
5' 6"	120-133	130-144	140-159
5' 7"	123-136	133-147	143-163
5' 8"	126-139	136-150	146-167
5' 9"	129-142	139-153	149-170
5' 10"	132-145	142-156	152-173
5' 11"	135-148	145-159	155-176
6' 0"	138-151	148-162	158-179

Weights at ages 25-59 based on lowest mortality. Weight in pounds according to frame (in indoor clothing weighing 3 lbs.; shoes with 1" heels).

Metropolitan Life Insurance height-weight chart for women.

Height and Weight Table For Men

Height	Small Frame	Medium Frame	Large Frame
5' 2"	128-134	131-141	138-150
5' 3"	130-136	133-143	140-153
5' 4"	132-138	135-145	142-156
5' 5"	134-140	137-148	144-160
5' 6"	136-142	139-151	146-164
5' 7"	138-145	142-154	149-168
5' 8"	140-148	145-157	152-172
5' 9"	142-151	148-160	155-176
5' 10"	144-154	151-163	158-180
5' 11"	146-157	154-166	161-184
6' 0"	149-160	157-170	164-188
6' 1"	152-164	160-174	168-192
6' 2"	155-168	164-178	172-197
6' 3"	158-172	167-182	176-202
6' 4"	162-176	171-187	181-207

Weights at ages 25-59 based on lowest mortality. Weight in pounds according to frame (in indoor clothing weighing 5 lbs.; shoes with 1" heels).

Metropolitan Life Insurance height-weight chart for men.

It's a good idea for you and your partner to get on the scale and record your starting weight. When you retest yourself, knowing where you started and how far you've come will be very inspiring.

Body Fat Composition

A better method for measuring body fat is by measuring your *body composition*. Body composition reflects the percentage of body fat as opposed to lean body mass (bone, muscle, tissue, blood, and organs). It is a more scientific and reliable measure of the physical condition you are in than the preceding scale method. There are a number of tests that produce your score; you will need the help of a professional fitness expert for most.

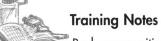

Training Notes

Body composition refers to the percentage of fat versus lean tissue in the body.

Cadaver Measurement

The truest measure of body composition is one that none of us want to ever go through. In this procedure, the body fat is cut away from the corpse and measured. We recommend you wait a while before you have this one performed. We hear it's really invasive and the plastic surgeons are not that good at repairing the scars.

Underwater Weighing

This is the "gold standard" of body composition testing, the test that the others strive to duplicate. You sit on an underwater scale, exhale all the air from your lungs, and then submerge yourself until your weight is recorded on the scale. Your underwater weight is then put into a formula that calculates your body composition. While this test is very accurate, it's not that comfortable, especially if you aren't fond of being submerged underwater.

Skinfold Measurements

Better known as the pinch test. The key to this test is to find a fitness professional who is proficient in this type of testing. There is a true science in knowing how to conduct this test the proper way. The fitness professional will take a number of "pinches" to measure the skin and fat. The numbers are then put into a formula and translated into your body composition.

Tape Measure Test

This test does not actually measure your body composition, but it does give a person an easy way to measure the number of inches lost around their body. The most common areas to measure include the neck, chest, arm, waist, hip, and thigh. You can even do it at home, just be sure that you are measuring the same anatomical locations test after test.

If you and your partner belong to a gym, chances are you'll be able to get your body fat measured by the skin fold test. Ask the staff if they are qualified to do this for you. The following chart shows the recommended ranges for men and women.

	Women	Men
Essential fat	10-12%	2-4%
Athletes	14-20%	6-13%
Fitness	21-24%	14-17%
Acceptable	25-31%	18-25%
Obese	32% plus	26% plus

The American Council of Exercise body fat percentage index.

If you are unable to get a skin fold test, you should do some tape measurements at the very least. You and your partner can measure each other. Record these numbers somewhere until it's time to measure again.

Cardiovascular Fitness

This is an area where you and your partner may improve the most, so you'll definitely want to do the test outlined here. While there are a wide range of tests a doctor or fitness professional can use to measure cardiovascular fitness, we've selected the Three-Minute Step Test because it's easy to administer and you and your partner can do it together, without the help of a professional.

This test is designed to measure your cardiovascular endurance. Using a 12-inch high bench (or a similarly sized stair in your house), step on and off for three minutes. Step up with one foot and then the other. Step down with one foot and then the other. Try to maintain a

steady four-beat cycle: "Up, up, down, down." At the end of three minutes, immediately check your heart rate by taking your pulse for one minute. Compare your result to the chart below.

3-Minute Step Test

3-Minute Step Test (Men)						
Age	18-25	26-35	36-45	46-55	56-65	65+
Excellent	<79	<81	<83	<87	<86	<88
Good	79-89	81-89	83-96	87-97	86-97	88-96
Above Average	90-99	90-99	97-103	98-105	98-103	97-103
Average	100-105	100-107	104-112	106-116	104-112	104-113
Below Average	106-116	108-117	113-119	117-122	113-120	114-120
Poor	117-128	118-128	120-130	123-132	121-129	121-130
Very Poor	>128	>128	>130	>132	>129	>190

3-Minute Step Test (Women)						
Age	18-25	26-35	36-45	46-55	56-65	65+
Excellent	<85	<88	<90	<94	<95	<90
Good	85-98	88-89	90-102	94-104	95-104	90-102
Above Average	99-108	0-111	103-110	105-115	105-112	103-115
Average	109-117	112-119	111-118	116-120	113-118	116-122
Below Average	118-126	120-126	119-128	121-129	119-128	123-128
Poor	127-140	127-138	129-140	127-135	129-139	129-134
Very Poor	>128	>138	>140	>135	>139	<134

Three-Minute Step Test chart.

Muscular Endurance

These are more easy tests for you and your partner to administer with each other. For evaluation purposes, muscular endurance is measured by a one-minute sit-up test and a push-up test. While these tests measure the endurance of the abdominal and chest muscles, they provide a good guesstimation of the muscular endurance in your entire body.

To perform the sit-up test, lie on the floor with your knees bent, feet flat. Your hands should rest on your thighs.

Squeeze your stomach, push your back flat, and raise high enough for your hands to touch the tops of your knees. Don't pull with your neck or head and keep your lower back on the floor. If you have back problems, it's okay to put your fingertips lightly on the back or your neck or head. Count how many sit-ups you can do in one minute and then check the chart for your rating.

1-Minute Sit-Up Test

1-Minute Sit-Up Test (Men)						
Age	18-25	26-35	36-45	46-55	56-65	65+
Excellent	>49	>45	>41	>35	>31	>28
Good	44-49	40-45	35-41	29-35	25-31	22-28
Above Average	39-43	35-39	30-34	25-38	21-24	19-21
Average	35-38	31-34	27-29	22-24	17-20	15-18
Below Average	31-34	29-30	23-26	18-21	13-16	14-Nov
Poor	25-30	22-28	17-22	13-17	12-Sep	10-Jul
Very Poor	<25	<22	<17	<9	<9	<7

1-Minute Sit-Up Test (Women)						
Age	18-25	26-35	36-45	46-55	56-65	65+
Excellent	>43	>39	>33	>27	>24	>23
Good	37-43	33-39	27-33	22-27	18-24	17-23
Above Average	33-36	29-32	23-26	18-21	13-17	14-16
Average	29-32	25-28	19-22	14-17	12-Oct	13-Nov
Below Average	25-28	21-24	15-18	13-Oct	9-Jul	10-May
Poor	18-24	13-20	14-Jul	9-May	6-Mar	4-Feb
Very Poor	<18	<20	<7	<5	<3	<2

One-Minute Sit-Up chart.

To perform the push-up test, men should use the standard "military style" push-up position with only the hands and the toes touching the floor. Women have the option of using the "bent knee" position. To do this, kneel on the floor, hands on either side of the chest, and keep your back straight. Do as many push-ups as possible until exhaustion. Count the total number of push-ups performed. Use the following chart to find out how you rate.

Push-Up Test

Push-Up Test (Men)						
Age	17-19	20-29	30-39	40-49	50-59	60-65
Excellent	>56	>47	>41	>34	>31	>30
Good	47-56	39-47	34-41	28-34	25-31	24-30
Above Average	35-46	30-39	25-33	21-28	18-24	17-23
Average	19-34	17-19	13-24	11-20	9-17	6-16
Below Average	11-18	10-16	8-12	6-10	5-8	3-5
Poor	4-10	4-9	2-7	1-5	1-4	1-2
Very Poor	<4	<4	<2	0	0	0

Push-Up Test (Women)						
Age	17-19	20-29	30-39	40-49	50-59	60-65
Excellent	>35	>36	>37	>31	>25	>23
Good	27-35	30-36	30-37	25-31	21-25	19-23
Above Average	21-27	23-29	22-30	18-24	15-20	13-18
Average	11-20	12-22	10-21	8-17	7-14	5-12
Below Average	6-10	7-11	5-9	4-7	3-6	2-4
Poor	2-5	2-6	1-4	1-3	1-2	1
Very Poor	0-1	0-1	0	0	0	0

One-Minute Push-Up chart.

Flexibility

Last but not least, there is flexibility. You may be tempted to skip this test because you think that flexibility is not that important to your overall fitness, but it is probably the most important of the three. As you age, your muscles lose their elasticity. Better to know what your flexibility level is and how much you need to work on it so you can still bend down and touch your toes when you're eighty!

To perform the flexibility test, sit on the floor with your feet shoulder-width apart, legs extended in front of you. Place your hands between your legs with your fingertips pointing toward your toes. Your partner can place a yardstick between your feet, positioning the edge of the stick next to your heels. Without bending your knees, hinge at your hips, reach forward with your hands, and touch as far up the yardstick as you can. Your partner will watch the number on the ruler that you touch and record that number. That number might not mean much to you now, but wait until you can reach three inches farther the next time!

We know that taking all of these measurements may not be high on your list of things to do, but trust us when we say you will be glad you did. Knowing where you started is important to knowing how far you've come.

Goal Setting

When you get to the point of goal setting, you and your partner need to have a lengthy discussion. After all, the purpose of your fitness union is to help each other meet your fitness goals. Setting goals gives you a plan for how you will design your fitness program, so don't skip this step. Would you build a house without a blueprint? Would you drive from Virginia to California without a map? We hope not! Consider what your personal goals are as well as what your partnership goals are. You should have long-term goals and short-term goals that you can measure and that are reasonably attainable. In this section, we outline the important steps to take and things to consider when you and your partner each define your goals.

SMART Goals

Remember the acronym of SMART Goals when you plan your fitness journey. A SMART goal is one that is Specific, Measurable, Attainable, Realistic, and Timely.

Specific

In order to achieve your goal, it must be well defined. To say, "I want to lose weight" is not very specific. How much weight do you want to lose? A more specific goal would be "I want to lose ten pounds." To help make your goal specific, try answering the "W" questions about it:

- ◆ **Who:** Who is involved in this goal?
- ◆ **What:** What is the end result of the goal?
- ◆ **When:** What is the time frame for achieving the goal (from the start of the goal to the end)?
- ◆ **Where:** Where will I pursue the goal?
- ◆ **Why:** Why am I pursuing the goal?
- ◆ **Which:** Which requirements or constraints do I need to be aware of as I pursue my goal?

Example: A general goal would be, "Get in shape." But a specific goal would be "Exercise with my friend Jim at the gym, and work out three days a week."

Measurable

What good is setting a goal if you don't know when you've achieved it? When you've completed your goal you should have some tangible evidence that you achieved success. It always feels good to have something in front of you to prove a job well done. This does not mean you need a trophy for every accomplishment. However, you should have some way to prove your success to yourself.

Example: A measurable goal would be "I want to run a 5K race in under thirty minutes."

Attainable

This is where some people run into a problem in the goal-setting process. Too often, people set goals that are just not within reach. What is the point of setting a goal that you can't achieve? You are just setting yourself up for failure and we don't want to see you get disappointed. Before you commit to your goal, make sure you have enough time and resources to accomplish it. If your goal is to be able to run a marathon, but you have chronic knee problems, your goal may not actually be attainable. Try something closer to your ability level.

Example: Completing a marathon might not be attainable if you've never even run around the block. A more attainable goal would be running a 5K race.

Realistic

Before you mention your goal to your partner, consider whether it is realistic. A realistic goal is one that is reasonable and sensible to commit to. Just because you truly want to achieve the goal doesn't mean it's realistic. All good intentions are met with unexpected obstacles. For example, your goal may be to work out every day of the week. You may really want to work out every day of the week, but do you think this is realistic? It's extremely likely that on any given day some unforeseen circumstance could stand in the way of your working out. Don't make the mistake of setting an unrealistic goal.

Example: "I will do some form of exercise at least four days per week."

Timely

All good goals have a time stamp. How long will it take you to achieve this goal? Without the time stamp, goals become less urgent, less important, and less of a factor in your life. Set a time limit for your goal and see how much harder you'll work to achieve it.

Example: "I want to lose ten pounds before my birthday in February."

With SMART goals you can succeed!

Partnership and Individual Goals

You and your partner may not have the same individual goals, but you can help each other by having a partnership goal. Often it is much harder to break a mutual goal with a partner than to break a goal with yourself. Your partner is counting on you, and you are counting on your partner to make your goal a commitment. Give your partner permission to hold you to your end of the goal. Here are some examples of partnership goals:

◆ We will go walking together at least three days per week for one hour.

◆ We will participate in one charity race event before the end of the year.

◆ We will improve our sit-up test scores by 20 percent in the next three months.

Partnership goals are important because they keep you both committed to each other and to the goals you set for your relationship. Accomplishing these partnership goals together will only improve the bond that you have.

Whatever your goal, remember to reward yourself for all of your hard work and commitment:

◆ If your goal was to be able to run a marathon, then go do it. Find a local race or plan a fitness vacation to another American or international city. There are dozens of marathons in almost every major city.

◆ If you are a woman and your goal was to drop two dress sizes, then go out and buy that new sexy and sleek outfit, maybe even something special for your "special partner."

◆ If you goal was to exercise three days a week for six months, then celebrate your success by taking a vacation, buying something you've wanted, or pampering yourself.

Remember that your fitness journey is just that, a journey. When driving from Virginia to California, you might want or need to take a detour. Let your fitness journey do the same thing. There is a path for your journey from beginning to end. If you wander from the path, don't let that bog you down, just get back on the path and continue to the end.

Establishing a Workout Schedule

Without a doubt, the most difficult part about your new fitness program is going to be finding the time to do it. It is, after all, the number one reason people give for not currently being involved in a fitness program. They just don't have the time. So the first challenge for you and your partner is making the time to exercise and making it a high enough priority so that you aren't always canceling your workouts for other things. The trick: Make an exercise appointment.

We've worked with hundreds of high-powered, high-stress, and very busy corporate, government, and organizational executives. The one thing that always amazes us is that even with their busy and confusing schedules, they always find time for exercise, either alone or with a partner. If these people can find time to exercise, so can you! Here are some suggestions:

- One of the real tricks of the trade is to consider your workout time as a business appointment. Put your workout in your daily schedule and let nothing take you away from it.

- Let those around you know about your fitness goal and remind them that they should treat your workout time like any other appointment. You need privacy and should not be interrupted.

- If you travel often, ask your travel agent to find a hotel that has an adequate fitness center or a location where you can be outside and exercise. Plan your exercise around your meetings and appointments while traveling.

- Hold your workout partner to your exercise appointment as well. If you are to meet Tuesday and Thursday at noon to exercise, make sure they have it on their calendar as well and don't take no for an answer.

- While keeping yourself and your partner on track, bear in mind that sometimes life does get in the way. Be flexible with your workouts and schedule. If you miss a workout due to a work emergency, don't let yourself get down. Maintain a positive attitude and strive to keep it from happening again.

Can I Get That in Writing?

You're more likely to stick with your exercise and your partnership if you put everything down in a contract. You'd be amazed at how much motivation a piece of paper listing the goals you've committed to reaching, signed by you, can provide. Hang a copy of your contract in places where you will see it often. Some good places include:

- **On your bathroom mirror**—You can look at it and review both in the morning and in the evening as you brush your teeth. Two minutes of focused attention on your goals!

- **On your refrigerator**—How many times do you make a trip to the fridge? Not only will you see your commitment every time, but it might also remind you *not* to go for the late-night snack or the leftovers.

- **On your computer screen**—Just tape it on your computer screen or television so that you are reminded of its importance and it might even motivate you to take a walk rather than watch TV or surf the web.

In addition to your contract, you might also want to include your goals and review them often.

The Least You Need to Know

◆ Defining your relationship with your partner will set the tone for productive and successful exercise sessions.

◆ Goals must be specific and attainable for each partner.

◆ Establishing a regular workout schedule with your partner will ensure long-term success.

◆ A fitness contract is a great way to form a strong commitment between both partners to reaching the goal.

In This Chapter

- ◆ Learn how to set the pace for every workout so you and your partner achieve maximum results

- ◆ Small changes that produce big results when your motivation starts to fade

- ◆ Using friendly competition to motivate your fitness partner

- ◆ How to overcome a plateau in your workout success

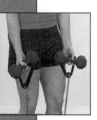
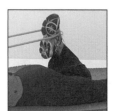
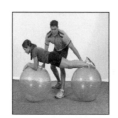
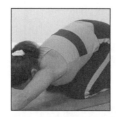
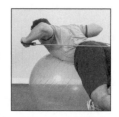
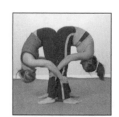

Chapter 4

Partner Pacing

If Chapter 3 was all about getting on the horse, then this chapter is about getting that horse to gallop. While that usually starts with cracking the whip, you've got to learn your partner's rhythm in order to help them keep the pace.

In this chapter, you'll find a list of tools to help keep you and your partner moving when your enthusiasm fades.

Know the Speed Limit

Every good driver is aware of a road's speed limit. While a speed limit on a given road is the same for every driver, we all know that each car handles differently under the same conditions. As the driver of your car, you learn how your car handles at certain speeds and in certain conditions. You learn how much pressure to apply on the brake, or how hard to turn the wheel. What happens when you drive someone else's car? It feels different, right?

The same principles apply to exercise and partner training. While you may know how fast you can accelerate through a workout, your partner's optimal performance pace may be different. Some days your engine may be sputtering while your partner's is all revved up. At other times, you'll be ready to put the pedal to the metal and your partner will be riding the brake. The trick is to find the speed limit that works for both of you on any given day.

This, of course, is easier said than done. One way to maximize the potential productivity of the exercise session is to set the pace of the workout before you begin. If you and your partner are both aware of the intensity level of the workout before you start, you may be able to better prepare for the effort you'll have to put forth. And while we realize that it will be a rare occasion that both of you will be up to the same level on the same day, sometimes just knowing what you are up against is all it takes to rev your engine.

Sunday Driving

Sunday drivers. Don't they always seem to be out on the road, inevitably right in front of you, just when you need to get somewhere in a hurry? They seem to be driving with no particular purpose. They're just out enjoying the road.

When you choose a Sunday Driving workout, you're essentially saying that you aren't looking to get anywhere quick, you're just along for the ride. Sunday Driving workouts are not designed to burn major calories, or even make you really sweat. They are just there to keep you moving. That's not to say they aren't important—they are. You need a Sunday Driving workout every now and then to allow your muscles an adequate recovery period and to remind yourself that exercise can be enjoyable.

Good examples of Sunday Driving workouts include:

- **Walking from garage sale to garage sale on a Saturday afternoon.** Even better if you make a few small purchases so you have an extra load to carry!
- **An easy hike to picnic at a campground.** (Of course you will pack a healthy picnic lunch!)
- **Playing a round of golf.** And no carts! You're walking these eighteen holes.
- **Gardening.** Disguise this workout as a fun day in the garden and you can discreetly sucker your partner into helping you pull weeds for hours on end. It doesn't sound like much of a workout, but just wait. You'll feel it the next day.

Fit Facts

Good times to incorporate a Sunday Driving workout into your schedule would be after a hard workout the day before, when you are short on time, or when you have met one of your fitness goals. The Sunday Driving workout can feel like a reward after a lot of hard work.

Indy Car Racing

The Indy Car pace is all out, pedal to the metal, full speed ahead. You stop for fuel, but only if you need it. You accelerate often to pass other cars and change lanes frequently to avoid getting stuck at the back of the pack. You hardly ever look in your rear view mirror except to marvel at the dust you've left in your wake. The Indy Car driver is concerned with one thing: speed.

If you choose an Indy Car pace for your workout, you had better be prepared to go until you run out of gas. That means high intensity, little rest, and short bursts of speed when you've got the energy. This type of workout is great for building endurance and stamina. Adding an Indy Car day once per week will help to keep your body guessing and is sure to prevent onset of the Dreaded Plateau. (More on that later in this chapter.)

Some ideas for Indy Car workouts include:

- **A stationary cycling class.** These classes are designed to combine shorts bursts of energy with periodic recovery periods. You'll definitely be out of gas when you finish.
- **Jumping rope.** Sounds elementary, until you get going. Jumping rope is a great total body aerobic activity. See how long you can go without stopping and then challenge yourself to beat that goal every time.

◆ **Sprints.** If you are a runner, consider doing a day of only sprints. After a brief warm-up, set up a series of sprint distances with short recovery periods in between. You won't be able to go as long, but your body will appreciate the wake-up call.

Workout Worries

The Indy Car workout should be incorporated into your workout plan when you feel you've developed adequate endurance and strength. Don't try the Indy Car workout in the first week of your program. Your body will respond better if you give yourself time to prepare for the challenge.

The Commuter

The commuter is the everyday driver experience. The destination is usually the same, with some shortcuts here and there. Occasionally you take a detour, which may lengthen your overall trip, but for the most part you're traveling in familiar territory. The commuter driver is looking to get to the destination in a respectable amount of time while avoiding tickets for speeding and other mishaps.

The Commuter workout, like commuter driving, is going to be your everyday workout experience. Occasionally you will add a little twist to keep you awake on the road, but for the most part you will know the routine well. The great thing about a commuter workout is that you will be able to jump right into the routine without a lot of thought or planning. This is great for those days when you just want to get in, get out, and sweat a little in between.

Fit Facts

The best workout plan will include at least one Sunday Driving and one Indy Car program per week. The remaining days can be your typical Commuter plan.

Great Commuter workouts combine the following:

◆ Thirty to sixty minutes of aerobic activity at sixty to eighty percent of your maximum heart rate.

◆ Thirty to sixty minutes of strength training, working all muscles to *muscular fatigue*.

◆ At least ten minutes of a stretching routine to include pilates or yoga exercises.

Training Notes

Muscular fatigue refers to the point at which a muscle achieves temporary exhaustion and can no longer overcome the overload placed on it.

Taking the Detour

Imagine that you are driving along the interstate when you come upon a car moving a little slower than you. You are not sure you want to risk passing them because that eager state trooper might be lurking around the bend. You decide to stay put. But after a while, you get bored staring at the same license plate in front of you. You're getting impatient. You want to take the next exit and follow the detour, don't you?

Let's change gears for a moment. (Yes, we're beating this driving analogy to death. We have a knack for that.) Snap back to your workout session with your partner. There may come a time when you two get stuck in a similar situation. You start to notice after several months that the scenery is not changing in your workout routine. Maybe you are starting to dread meeting each other at 6:30 A.M. at the gym because it means you'll run into the same people in the parking lot, in the locker room, and in the fitness center. This means one thing. You've become what's called "a regular" and you're not really liking it. So what are you going to do? Take the detour!

You definitely want to take the road less traveled. You've got to break free of the monotony of your routine or you will lose motivation and excitement. More importantly, if you keep things the way they are, you'll start to notice you aren't making as much progress as you once were. For these reasons and more, take the detour!

Workout Worries

If you notice that your enthusiasm for your exercise program fades as you face another day of the same old fitness routine, make a change that day. Don't wait. A small change in your program could mean a big change in your results.

Common scenery-changing maneuvers:

- **Head Outdoors.** If you normally meet at the gym every morning, consider meeting at a local park for a few weeks. Adopting an outdoor exercise routine will not only help break the routine, but being outdoors will invigorate your senses and leave you feeling energized.

Workout Worries

Taking your exercise outdoors may do more than just break your routine. Experts believe that exposure to sunlight and fresh air while exercising may enhance your overall exercise experience. Mental health experts believe that connecting with nature can create a calming effect while medical experts report that exposure to the outdoors increases Vitamin D production. All great reasons to take it outside!

- **Blaze a New Trail.** Do you always walk or run the same route? Try going a different way every day for a week. You and your partner can take turns choosing the route. No doubt you'll cure the boredom and find some great new sites to see.

- **Take a Lesson.** Always wanted to learn to play tennis but don't even own a racket? Considering getting involved in group lessons one night per week. If the activity is new and different, chances are you will look forward to attending. Trying out a new sport can motivate you and make you feel like a kid again.

- **Start at the End.** Do you typically start every workout session with your aerobic activity, then move to weight training and stretching? Try mixing that up. After a short warm-up, do your strength-training exercises first. With more energy at the start of the workout, you may be able to work a little harder on the weights, which could translate into big strength gains.

- **Get Some Class.** Aerobic class, that is. If you've been hesitant to try a new group exercise class at the gym, now would be a good time to sample it. Finding a great class with an excellent instructor can really give you something to look forward to, even if it's only one time per week.

And doing this with your partner will give you the support and encouragement you may need at that first class.

Workout Worries

If you are hesitant to participate in a group exercise class, talk to the instructor. Let her know that you're a beginner and ask what the overall fitness level of the class is. If this class is too advanced, ask her to recommend another that you could start out in.

The Competitive Edge

Imagine standing at the start line of a big race. You've trained for months for this moment. Your emotions are running the gamut and you hope that your months of training pay off and you cross the finish line triumphantly. If this thought does not scare you to death, you've got a competitive side in you just itching to get out.

Entering a competition, whether a race or something else, can tremendously enhance the level of everyday training for you and your partner. First it requires that you commit to competing together. By doing so, you are making a promise to your partner that you will help them meet this goal and that you will succeed together. Second, entering this competition most likely means that you will adopt a new training program designed to help you meet this specific goal. Having a target training program means new workout challenges for you and your partner. And third, training for a competition means that you will have to be dedicated in order to succeed. You can't succeed if you don't prepare. Just knowing that a competition is on the horizon and that you have to train in order to complete it will motivate you to stay dedicated to your exercise plan, even when you want to slack off for just one day.

Don't Sweat It

Not sure about competitive events in your area? Or are you considering traveling to your fitness event? The Internet is full of websites for different competitions. These websites often include information about the actual event, as well as travel, accommodations, and local points of interest. Considering planning your next vacation around a race event.

Need more reasons to try a competition? Consider these:

- **The Charity.** Most local events are sponsored by a charity, with proceeds going to support that charity. By entering a charity competition, you are not only bettering yourself, but you're potentially helping someone else along the way. The larger charitable organizations even provide training support for athletes who raise money for their cause.

- **The T-Shirt.** No kidding. Almost all events include receipt of a commemorative T-shirt. Don't knock it. We know you could use an extra workout shirt. When was the last time you washed yours anyway?

- **The Trophy.** Not all, but some events give medals or trophies to participants. And let's be honest, who doesn't need an extra trophy to add to their collection? You can put it on the shelf next to your runner-up spelling bee trophy from third grade.

The decision to enter a competition should be a careful one. Consider your and your partner's strengths, interests, and training abilities. Maybe endurance activities are not your strong point, but strength competitions are right up your alley. The idea of a body-building competition might have you laughing now, but think about it again after a few months with your fitness program. Watch out, Arnold!

When you select an event, give yourselves plenty of time to train for it. In order to feel comfortable on the big day, you have to feel prepared. And lastly, choose something fun! There are lots of great events out there that focus more on the camaraderie than the competition.

The Dreaded Plateau

All of the ideas we've shared in this chapter are designed to help you avoid the exercise *plateau*. No doubt you've heard this term before. It's that exercise purgatory that kills your momentum and squashes your motivation. It's the roadblock in your journey toward physical fitness that seems impossible to detour around.

What is a plateau in exercise terms? It is the point in your program at which you stop making progress and can only maintain your current level of fitness.

The plateau is frustrating because it strikes without warning. Usually you are experiencing a very high level of success with your program when it hits. You're rolling along, losing weight, building endurance, feeling great, and then, Whammo! The plateau.

> **Training Notes**
>
> A **plateau** is any period in development where neither progress nor decline takes place.

Although the plateau is often an unwelcome invasion into your exercise plan, you should heed it as a warning sign. What is your exercise plateau trying to tell you? Let's look at possible messages and how to respond.

Not Enough Energy

What do you mean not enough energy? You've been feeling great for weeks! But in this case, we're not talking mental energy, we're talking food energy. Here's the deal: It takes calories to burn calories. When you decrease your food intake, your body simply lowers its metabolic rate in response. This allows the body to function but creates hunger and prevents you from losing fat. This is also called the "starvation mode."

The best way to tackle this is to keep your caloric intake slightly below your metabolic needs. That way, you keep the pump primed, so to speak, giving your body enough of what it needs to work, without flooding it out.

Weight Loss

This one is going to hurt: Your very goal of losing weight may cause you to stop losing weight. How's that for cruel and unusual punishment?

The problem is that weight loss naturally lowers your metabolism. As you lose weight, the body requires less energy to maintain its functions. If you lose too much too quickly, your body will respond with a plateau to safeguard against a total breakdown.

The best way to deal with this kind of plateau is to increase your strength-training regime. This will help to increase your lean body mass. Don't be dismayed if that scale doesn't show that you're losing more weight. With this trick, you'll be losing body fat, and that's even better.

The Honeymoon Is Over

By honeymoon, we're referring to the *adaptation phase* of your workout program. In this phase, your body records the most significant physiological changes because it is responding to the increase in demand that you have just placed on it. After a while though, it will make adjustments and begin to burn fewer calories with the same amount of effort.

Training Notes

The **adaptation phase** of a workout refers to the first several weeks when your body is making several adjustments to the increase in demands. Its response is evidenced by a significant physiological change in a short period of time. The length of the adaptation phase is different for different people. You'll know when you hit that plateau that the honeymoon is over.

The solution to this problem is to continually change your exercise program. We've given you a lot of great ideas in this chapter for staying motivated and introducing change into your workout. The key is to challenge the body to continue to adapt.

Overtraining

Some folks get excited about their new exercise adventure and dive in too deep too quickly. If that concept makes you laugh, then you might be one of these people. However, when you exercise too much, your body can reach a point of diminishing returns. At this point, your body is rejecting your efforts to improve itself. You have essentially made your body mad.

Most people think that as long as they are exercising, they will continue to build muscle. However, when you exercise, you are actually breaking down the muscle fibers. The building takes place during the rest period when the body repairs the damaged muscle fibers and recruits more fibers for the next exercise session. When you don't allow for recovery, the muscle does not have time to rebuild and the improvements that you were noticing at first will start to diminish.

The solution to this problem is easy: Take a break. The body needs time for recovery and rest. Take a break from exercise for a couple days or try a Sunday Driving workout and enjoy the change.

If you understand the source of your plateau, you can take immediate steps to reverse it. The worst thing you can do is ignore your plateau. If you let it go too long, you could become discouraged by your lack of progress and lose motivation or you could end up with an injury if overtraining is to blame. The best way to overcome the plateau is to expect it.

The Least You Need to Know

◆ Setting the pace for each workout session before you start will ensure that both you and your partner are prepared for the challenge.

◆ Changing activities often will reduce the chance of boredom and help to maintain your motivation and enthusiasm for your goals.

◆ Adjusting your calorie intake can counterbalance any energy deficits you experience from your increased activity.

◆ The exercise plateau is a common predicament in most people's workout programs. Learn the source of yours and take steps to overcome it.

In This Chapter

- How to become more aware of the food choices you make and how they affect your body

- Tricks for avoiding the fat traps in common snacks

- Making food fun with your fitness partner

- Choosing food for fitness

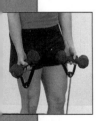
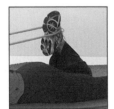
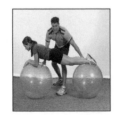
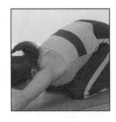
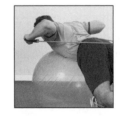
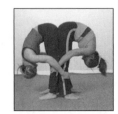

Chapter 5

Your Nutrition Team

Since we've got you making changes with your exercise habits, we thought we'd keep the momentum and throw in a chapter about your diet, too. Yes, diet—that ugly four-letter word. You see, your healthy new lifestyle doesn't end when you finish your workout. Not a chance. It's called a lifestyle because it affects every aspect of your life, including the food choices you make.

In this chapter, we're going to review some basic nutrition concepts, teach you how to support your partner when it comes to making healthy food choices, and illustrate some tricks for sneaking in treats when you really need them. So grab a bag of popcorn (the low-fat kind!) and read on as we decode the mystery of the diet.

Being the Food Police

Generally speaking, when people are surrounded by healthy food choices, they are more likely to choose those foods than their unhealthy counterparts. The same goes for the company you keep. Teaming up for nutrition is a great way to work on healthy food choices and consumption. Just think … how would you feel eating a burger and fries while your partner was eating a grilled salmon salad? Not only would you feel guilty, but your body wouldn't appreciate it as well.

It is important to work on nutrition with a partner. You will acknowledge each other's accomplishments and keep each other motivated. Here are the most important steps to changing your eating habits:

◆ **Write down everything you eat.** Show it to your partner, and have your partner show their list to you. Make it a competition to see who can eat healthier. The object is not to eat *nothing*, but to eat the right amounts of the right foods. Even though no one saw you sneak those extra cookies after lunch, your body knows.

◆ **Do like your mom told you, and eat your fruits and vegetables.** These foods are the most underrated and are the hidden secrets to your fitness success. Not only do they taste great, you can do almost anything with them, they are very low in calories, and packed with vitamins and minerals that you need to keep you healthy and well!

◆ **Understand that not everyone needs the same amount of food.** If you are 5'4", and your partner is 6'3", you probably don't need to eat as much as your partner. Choosing the same types of foods is a great idea, especially if you have the same tastes for food, but portion sizes are key to keeping your calories down.

◆ **Fad diets are just that—fads.** Falling into the schemes of fad diets will only prolong your goal of health and fitness. While many "diets" encompass healthy ideas, most are too extreme for you to stay on for long periods of time, and most lack something that your body needs to function at its highest capacity.

◆ **Be a trendsetter, not a follower.** When dining with your partner, friend, colleague, or family members, it is important to remember that, especially if they do not have the same goals in mind that you do, you need to make food choices on your own. Ultimately, it is your choice what you put into your body!

◆ **Keep trigger foods out of grasp.** If it's not around, it can't be eaten. If you know that when there's a bag of potato chips around, you are probably going to eat half the bag, stay as far away from potato chips as possible. Buy foods that are easy for you to control yourself around.

◆ **Learn to read food labels.** Food labels really do tell you what is in what you are eating. Look at the portion size first—many times this is ignored and can cause you to consume more calories than you had intended. Take into account not only the total amount of fat, but the type of fat (limit saturated fats). How much sodium is in the frozen entrée you are about to put in the microwave?

If your workout partner is your significant other, ever consider making a grocery date? What better way to show your love than by making healthy food choices as you walk (see, you even get added cardio benefits as well) the grocery store aisles? Don't forget to stop by the dairy counter and pull out a gallon of milk for your bicep curls!

Avoiding the Fat Trap

We need to listen to our bodies more often; the foods that usually cause us discomforts are high fat, high calorie, and high sodium foods. *Fat* hides in many foods, especially in prepared foods bought at stores and restaurants. An innocent bowl of soup or a "healthy" salad can contain up to 30 grams of fat and over 400 calories. Not all fats are created equally, though. Your body does need a certain amount of fat to function properly. Let's look at the different types of fat.

Training Notes

Fats are used to keep your body tissues insulated, transport fat-soluble vitamins throughout the body, and store energy.

◆ **Monounsaturated Fatty Acids:** These are the simplest forms of fats. They are liquid at room temperature, and found in vegetable oils such as olive oil, canola oil, and peanut oil. This type of fat, when ingested, may lower your LDL cholesterol levels and decrease your risk for cardiovascular disease.

◆ **Polyunsaturated Fatty Acids:** You can find these types of fat in seafood and vegetable oils including flaxseed, sunflower, safflower, and corn.

◆ **Saturated Fatty Acids:** Too much saturated fat can cause increases in LDL cholesterol levels and total cholesterol levels, and increase your risk of cardiovascular disease. Saturated fats are mainly found in animal products including poultry, meat, dairy products, and butter. These fats are solid at room temperature.

◆ **Trans Fatty Acids:** These fats are found in commercially packaged foods such as cookies, crackers, and fried foods. Look for "partially hydrogenated vegetable oil" or "shortening" in the ingredient list to spot these types of fats since it is not currently required by law for manufacturers to list how much is in foods. Trans Fats can raise LDL levels and lower HDL levels.

The goal is to stick with the 30 percent limit on fats. Thirty percent of what? Thirty percent of your total caloric intake. Broken down, your goal is:

◆ 10–15 percent of total calories from monounsaturated fat

◆ 10 percent of total calories from polyunsaturated fat

◆ 7–10 percent of total calories from saturated fat

To do this, choose foods that are generally low (not necessarily fat-free) in fat. Eat lots of fruits, vegetables, whole grains, and lean protein, and watch what is being put into your food. One way you can do this is by familiarizing yourself with certain cooking terms so you can make choices that will help you eliminate hidden fat.

Following are two lists. The first list contains cooking methods to help you limit your fat intake. Choose from it often. The second contains methods you should choose less often. (Remember—never deprive yourself of any food; moderation is key!)

"Healthy" Food Preparation Terms:

Bake: Food cooked in an oven surrounded by dry heat at a specific temperature.

Blanch: To shock raw vegetables in ice-cold water after briefly boiling them.

Broil: Food cooked directly under or over a heat source.

Grill: Food cooked over coals or other heat source.

Sauté: Food cooked in a small amount of oil or fat at a high temperature so that the food does not absorb too much of the oil.

Steam: To cook food over boiling liquid.

Stir-fry: To cook small amounts of food at a high heat in a wok or pan; food is stirred constantly to prevent burning.

"Less Healthy" Food Preparation Terms:

A la king: Diced foods served in a cream sauce.

Aioli sauce: Cold egg and olive oil emulsion with garlic.

Alfredo: A sauce containing butter, cream, and Parmesan cheese.

Bard: A lean meat with fat tied around it to keep it moist.

Béchamel sauce: A white sauce made with cream and thickened with roux.

Bisque: Cream-based soup.

Deep fry: Food is completely submerged in oil or fat that is held on an average at 375 degrees.

Florentine: Foods cooked with spinach and usually a cream sauce.

Hollandaise sauce: Warm egg and oil emulsion sauce.

Milanes: Food dipped in egg, breadcrumbs, and Parmesan cheese, then fried.

Remoulade: Mayonnaise-based French sauce.

Roux: Flour and fat used to thicken sauces, soups, and stews.

A Healthy Recipe Exchange and Other Fun Games

Not sure what to make for dinner now that you've turned over the health leaf? We all enjoy a good game here and there—why not make your new nutrition challenge a fun game to play alone or with your partner?

◆ Start looking for recipes. Look everywhere … magazines, the Internet, TV (There is the Cooking Network, of course!). Now that you've found all of these fabulous recipes, it's time to start sharing the health. You can do this with your partner, your colleagues, and your family members. The more recipes you have, the more options you have. Eating healthy means eating smart, not eating boring food! There are plenty of ways to dress up skinless, boneless chicken breast and broccoli.

◆ See how many recipes you and your partner can collect together. Then put them together and make your very own cookbook. Not only will it be beneficial to you and your partner, but you can give these away as presents to your friends and family. They will all appreciate your concern for their health and be impressed by your creativity.

◆ Another fun game you can play with your partner is one I like to call "Ready, Set, Go." Write down five goals that you don't think your partner is accomplishing nutrition-wise on a daily basis. Your partner will do the same. The game is to then see who can accomplish more of the five challenges and stick with it for seven full days. The person who doesn't accomplish as many goals must treat the winner to a healthy meal. (You can buy it or cook it, but it must be healthy!)

Celebrate Willpower!

So you've kept yourself under control and avoided the muffins for breakfast and the French fries for lunch. How do you reward yourself? First off, bring your partner along to help you celebrate. This way, you have someone there with you so that you don't "over"-celebrate. Choose your means of celebration wisely; it does not necessarily have to be food. You can choose to go shopping with your partner, go to the spa, or buy tickets to a show/sporting event. The point is, even though you've done well with food, you don't need to reward yourself with it.

If you are going to reward yourself with food, pick a designated day during the week. Also pick a designated food. If you usually eat ice cream every night for dinner, but have eliminated it completely, allow yourself one night a week to have one serving of ice cream. If you go out for dinner on Saturday nights and would like to splurge on that one night and have a pasta dish, watch your portion size and have lots of vegetables with it to fill you up.

Make sure you are doing this as a reward for the hard work you have done the rest of the week. Add your partner in this celebration and make it a party for two. Remember to compromise and make your reward something for both of you. This will give you both more incentive to keep up the good work without depriving yourself of your favorite foods. Being healthy is not about punishing yourself—it's about making smart choices and moderation.

With so much information in the media about fad diets and research being done, it's difficult for consumers to know what really needs to be done in order to eat healthy. Here are the top 10 basic rules that will help you sort through the mess of fact or fiction.

1. Eat Your Fruits and Vegetables.

Not only are they low in calories and high in flavor, but they will fill you up because they are loaded with fiber, vitamins, and minerals.

2. Drink Water. Lots of It.

Water has many functions in the body. The most obvious is hydration. Water also helps us flush out excess vitamins and minerals that our body doesn't need. It also helps us filter and process protein through the kidneys. Water keeps your skin moist and your hair shiny. Aim for six to eight eight-ounce glasses per day.

3. There Is No Such Thing as a Bad Food ... Moderation, Moderation.

If you deprive yourself of something completely, the likelihood that you are going to end up eating it (and probably overeating it) is inevitable. All foods have some sort of function. Some foods are just more nutritionally dense, which is why they are considered "healthier" for you. The important thing is to have control over your eating and food choices. All food can fit into your diet somewhere!

4. Eat Breakfast.

This really is the most important meal of the day. Not only will it give you needed energy for the rest of the day, but it can help prevent overeating during the remainder of the day.

5. Don't Skip Meals.

Skipping meals is a surefire way to end up overeating at the next meal. Eat small, frequent meals, and learn the difference between your body being hungry and just having "cravings."

6. Watch for Hidden Calories.

Hidden calories can be the difference between weight loss and gain. Most calories hide in sauces—whether it's mayonnaise, Aioli, or Hollandaise. This can turn an otherwise healthy meal into a caloric disaster.

7. Know Your Carbohydrates.

Carbohydrates have gotten a bad rap over the last 10 years. The important thing to realize is that not all carbohydrates are created equally.

Fruits and vegetables are considered carbohydrates, and eating these foods is not going to make you fat. Other carbohydrates include breads, pastas, rice, grains, and legumes. If you want to categorize any foods as "bad" carbohydrates, they are the foods made out of refined flour like white breads, pastas, and rice. These are not actually bad foods; they are not, however, as nutrient-dense as whole grains.

8. Eat Fewer Empty-Calorie Liquid Foods.

If you are trying to cut calories, one of the first and easiest ways to do it is to look at what you are drinking. Specialty coffee drinks, juice, and soda contain loads of calories and very little of anything else. Switch to water!

9. Go Grocery Shopping.

It is important to keep healthy food around so that you have no excuses. You will eat what you buy, so make smart choices while shopping. Choose lots of fresh fruits and vegetables, and healthy snacks like low-fat popcorn. Forget about the junk food—if it's not on your shelves, how can you eat it?

10. Bottom Line—Calories In vs. Calories Out.

Your weight depends on how many calories you take in compared to how many calories you use during the day. This includes normal day-to-day activities such as sitting, walking, talking, breathing, and sleeping, as well as exercise. If you take in more calories than your body uses in a day, those extra calories can add up to extra weight. So how do we combat putting on those extra pounds? The answer is not starving ourselves—it is to become more physically active and use moderation when making choices about food consumption.

Don't Sweat It

Did you know that one pound is equal to 3,500 calories?

The Least You Need to Know

◆ Just as with exercise, making a change in your nutrition habits takes time and dedication. With the help of your partner, this should be a "piece of cake."

◆ Don't deprive yourself of the food you crave. The key is moderation.

◆ Remember that many times there are different food choices that can make what you eat a bit healthier. You won't even notice a change in taste, just a change in your waistline.

In This Part

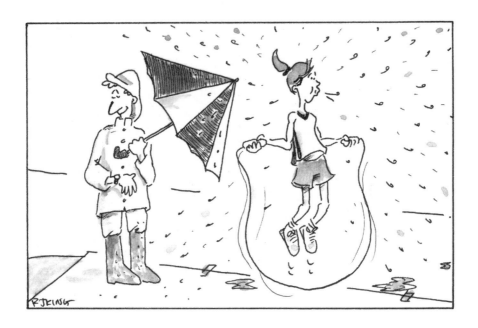

Part 2

Gonna Make You Sweat

A workout is twenty-five percent perspiration and seventy-five percent determination. Stated another way, it is one part physical exertion and three parts self-discipline. Doing it is easy once you get started.

—George Allen

Sweat is the evidence of hard work and determination. It's the badge of honor you wear after every workout to show that you gave it your all and you are coming back for more. Sweat illustrates that you know what it takes to achieve fitness success and that you won't give up without a fight.

The goal of this section is to make you sweat. Are you and your partner ready for your introduction to aerobic workouts and cardiovascular conditioning? Are you and your partner ready to find out if you have what it takes to get fit from the inside out? Are you and your partner ready to challenge your bodies to run more, bike more, jump more, and sweat more?

If you're sweating as you read this, don't worry. Sweat happens!

In This Chapter

- What is aerobic exercise?

- How aerobic exercise can improve your overall health

- What types of exercises are considered aerobic

- How to overcome your fear of aerobics

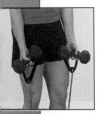
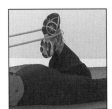
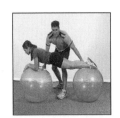
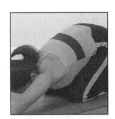
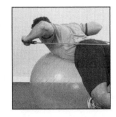
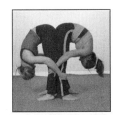

Chapter 6

Aerobiphobia

Aerobics. Just the word makes you feel a little funny inside. Maybe you conjure up images of leotards and Jane Fonda videos. Or maybe the image of Richard Simmons "sweatin' to the oldies" is forever burned in your mind. Whatever the case, you should know that the term aerobics doesn't only refer to an exercise class where you don leg warmers and jazzercise your way to total fitness.

In this chapter, we discuss the concept of aerobics and the types of exercise that are "aerobic" in nature. We will highlight how to overcome your fears of group exercise classes, negotiating the treadmill, and how to learn to love to sweat. We will also discuss why aerobic exercise is a key component of your workout program.

Keep turning the pages! It's time to sweat it out!

Aerobics

Before we go any further, we need to set the record straight about *aerobics*. Aerobics refers to the body systems that are being used to complete the exercise. But what does that mean?

Dr. Kenneth Cooper introduced the term aerobics in a 1968 book named, you guessed it, *Aerobics*. Dr. Cooper is a pioneer in exercise research and is credited with motivating more people to exercise and maintain their health than any other individual in the field. With aerobics, Dr. Cooper's mission was to steer the field of medicine away from disease treatment and toward disease prevention through aerobic exercise. His message: "It is easier to maintain good health through proper exercise, diet, and emotional balance than it is to regain it once it is lost."

Fit Facts

Dr. Kenneth Cooper has led the way in aerobic research since he wrote his first book titled *Aerobics* in 1968. Dr. Cooper is credited with leading more people toward a healthier lifestyle than any other individual in the fitness industry.

Dr. Cooper defined aerobic exercise as any activity that requires oxygen to perform. Activities that use large muscle groups, are rhythmic, and can be maintained continuously for long periods of time are considered to be aerobic. Since this clearly describes many group exercise classes, is not surprising that the term aerobic became synonymous with images of Jane Fonda and Richard Simmons. However, we want to break that stereotype right here and paint a friendlier picture of aerobic exercise. Your new thoughts of aerobics should include things like walking, running, and bicycling at a challenging yet comfortable pace.

Training Notes

Aerobic activity is any activity that uses large muscle groups, is rhythmic, and can be maintained continuously for long periods of time.

Why Should I Aerobicize?

So why all the fuss about aerobic exercise? As it turns out, aerobic activity is responsible for more physiological changes in the body than any other form of exercise. Take a look.

Aerobic activity …

◆ **Increases cardiovascular endurance.** Aerobic exercise conditions the heart, lungs, and cardiovascular system to process and deliver oxygen more expeditiously to every part of the body. As the heart muscle becomes stronger and more efficient, it can pump more blood to the muscles with each stroke requiring fewer strokes to effectively fuel the body. Therefore, an aerobically conditioned individual can work longer, more vigorously, and achieve a quicker recovery than her nonconditioned counterparts.

◆ **Increases metabolism.** We bet you like the sound of this already. During exercise, the metabolic rate is elevated to accommodate the increased demand on the body systems. With aerobic exercise, this metabolic rate remains elevated for several hours after the exercise session has ended, which can mean great calorie-burning effects for you. So in order to keep your metabolism up even when at rest, do more aerobics!

◆ **Reduces your risk of depression and anxiety.** Aerobic activity increases your body's secretion of endorphins, a hormone related to mood elevation (see Chapter 2). Increasing the release of endorphins into the bloodstream has been linked to decreasing the incidence of depression and anxiety-related disorders. As a matter of fact, many mental health professionals are prescribing aerobic activity as their first line of defense to combat depression-related illnesses.

◆ **Decreases blood pressure.** Hypertension, or high blood pressure, is associated with many cardiovascular-related diseases. Many studies have already shown that people who engage in aerobic activity have lower blood pressure than those who don't. And, unlike some drugs used to lower blood pressure, the side effects of exercise are generally only positive.

◆ **Reduces body fat.** Besides giving you a more toned and fit looking figure, reducing your total body fat can also reduce your risk of developing other medical problems including cardiovascular disease and diabetes. Aerobic activity is responsible for burning excess calories that would otherwise be stored in the body and contribute to weight gain. While the experts recommend at least 30 minutes of aerobic activity, any amount of exercise is better than none for reducing body fat and your risk of disease.

◆ **Reduces the risk of cardiovascular disease and diabetes.** Improving your overall fitness and decreasing your body fat can only improve your chances of steering clear of cardiovascular-related illnesses. The heart is a muscle like any other in the body. When it is strengthened through regular aerobic exercise, it is better equipped to ward off illness and diseases. A strong heart is a healthy heart.

Aerobic activity can impact every aspect of your physical health, from the way you look to the way you feel. Starting an aerobic exercise program at any age and any fitness level can produce almost immediate and lasting effects on your body. So don't delay one second longer. (Okay, maybe you can delay just a few more minutes to finish this chapter!)

But We Hate to Sweat

This is a common response from new exercisers. After all, there is a whole commercial market of personal products designed to prevent you from sweating in the first place, so why would you encourage such an offensive reaction in your body? Well, let us be the first to tell you that there is nothing wrong with a little sweat in your system. Sweat is your body's way of regulating its thermostat. Without a little sweat, you're

likely to overheat, and believe us when we tell you that you'd rather sweat a little than suffer from heat exhaustion. It's just not fun.

Fit Facts

Did you know that the average adult loses about 0.7 liters of sweat per day? And sweat losses from exercise can be as much as 2.5 liters per hour.

While we're on the subject, now would be a good time to address the "sweat factor" with your fitness partner. Not sure what the "sweat factor" is? Picture this—you're at the gym one day and the guy next to you on the treadmill is huffing and puffing away. At first you only feel a sprinkle. Then you are practically being rained on. This is an exaggeration, but you've seen this guy. You don't know what to make of this display of bodily dysfunction but you know you want to take shelter quickly.

Before you run for cover, keep in mind what we mentioned earlier: Sweat is your body's way of regulating its thermostat. However, not everybody's thermostat is running at the same level. So you will find that some people sweat more than others. This has nothing to do with fitness level. You could be superfit and sweat like a pig, and that's perfectly normal. The trick is to be aware of your sweat factor and how to manage it to keep everyone in your immediate surroundings comfortable.

Here are a few "Sweatiquette" tips to keep everyone happy and dry:

◆ **Always carry a sweat towel with you when in the gym.** Even if you aren't a really big sweater, carrying a towel shows your fellow gym goers and your fitness partner that you are trying your best to keep a clean environment.

- **If you are an excessive sweater, consider bringing several shirts to your workout.** Once a shirt is soaked, you'll leave a mark everywhere you go. Changing your shirt will freshen your look and keep everyone around you happy, too.

- **Be aware of body odor.** There is no faster way to scare off your partner than with a bad case of BO. Try the defensive approach with this one. Find a strong deodorant and apply liberally. Trust us. Deodorant is always a crowd pleaser!

- **Don't recycle your workout clothes.** We beg you. Workout clothes should be worn once and washed. While we'd like to think we don't need to point this out, we know we do. Just because you think you didn't sweat that much and can wear the shirt again, we promise you, you can't! Make it a habit to wash after every wear, just like your mother taught you.

Workout Worries

You may notice that while your partner is barely glistening after an hour-long workout, you have lost enough water to fill a bucket. Don't worry or be embarrassed. Just keep a towel with you and wipe down yourself and the equipment you are using often.

But We're Uncoordinated

There is another misconception out there in the mysterious world of the fitness unknown that says that you must be coordinated to participate in aerobic activity. While we will agree that many aerobic style classes are choreographed and can involved complicated steps, we have already said that exercise classes are not the only form of aerobic activity. So before you and your partner claim two left feet and shy away from aerobics all together, maybe you can try some of these other, less traditional, aerobic classes.

- **Boot Camp.** Sounds like fun, right? These classes are designed with the idea of military basic training in mind. The moves are simple and uncomplicated, allowing you to focus on the actual exercise and not on keeping your feet untangled. Boot camp classes are great to do with a partner because you can cheer each other on as you go through the drills. After all, the military loves a good sense of brotherhood.

- **Spinning.** Stationary cycling classes, also known as Spinning, are a fantastic aerobic workout. Participants pedal on their own stationary cycles as the instructor guides them through visualization exercises. Best thing: All you have to do is pedal!

- **Cardio Boxing.** Float like a butterfly, sting like a bee! We'll agree that Muhammad Ali was beautifully coordinated, but you don't need his skills to participate in today's cardio boxing classes. These classes mostly involve punch sequences designed to elevate your heart rate but keep you on your feet.

- **Interval Training.** Interval training classes are similar to boot camp-style classes in that the exercises are mostly basic in nature. The purpose of an interval class is to vary the intensity within the workout to combine periods of high intensity with periods of rest and recovery. Interval training is a great way to increase your endurance and prevent boredom.

Don't forget, aerobics is not all about exercise classes. Aerobics is about exercising the large muscle groups in the body. Here are some other forms of aerobic activity that you and your partner can do together.

- Walking
- Bicycling
- Swimming
- Kayaking
- Hiking
- Jumping Rope

Okay, so maybe jumping rope requires a little bit of coordination, but a few turns of the rope and you'll get the hang of it!

But We're Afraid of the Treadmill

Okay, now you're reaching for excuses here. We realize that some exercise machines can be intimidating with all of their moving parts and electronic displays. It seems that every year more and more gadgets are added to these machines to try to distract you from the fact that you still have to do the work when you get on them. Some machines even have computers attached to them so you can surf the web or play video games while you exercise. Like a treadmill wasn't scary enough. Then they go and add a plasma TV screen to it to really frighten you.

Whatever the case, gadgets or no gadgets, we realize that your first time on an exercise machine with moving parts can be a little bit stressful. Lucky for you, you have a partner who may be able to show you the ropes. Even if your partner is just as intimidated as you are, then you can both support each other as you tackle the monstrous machinery in your gym.

Our suggestion is to get a thorough orientation of all of the equipment by a qualified staff member before you test anything out. They will be able to show you how to turn it on, as well as any safety concerns that you may need to consider. Don't skip out on the orientation if you've never used the equipment before. You could be cheating yourselves out of a safe and effective workout.

So what happens if you go through the orientation and still have a small mishap when you step on the treadmill? You need to learn the art of the graceful recovery. It goes something like this: As the treadmill belt is spinning you around like a towel in the spin cycle of a washing machine, wait patiently until it eventually shoots you off the back. Then stand slowly, brush yourself off, and promptly throw your hands in the air like an Olympic gymnast finishing her dismount. This is sure to get some applause from your partner and any onlookers!

Don't Sweat It

It is rare that people injure themselves on equipment when they are at the gym. However, it is possible and you should know what to do if it happens to you. First, report it to a staff member immediately. While you may be embarrassed and not want to call additional attention to yourself, it is important to let someone know that you did fall, even if you are not visibly injured. Second, get medical attention if you are injured. Do not ignore your injuries, even if they are minor scrapes. Gym equipment is crawling with bacteria and one open wound can easily lead to an infection. Third, follow up with the gym staff if other problems develop. Some injuries do not surface immediately. If you notice pain or discomfort even several days after the accident, let the staff know. Lastly, get back on the horse. Don't let one bad experience keep you from getting back on that machine.

But We Don't Need to Lose Weight

Congratulations! You are part of a small group of people who didn't begin an exercise program to lose weight. While you are a minority, we know your reasons for beginning to exercise with a partner are important and we applaud your commitment to your overall health. If you are committed to continuing to improve your fitness level even though you don't need to lose weight, then you will certainly understand that aerobic activity is not just a fat-burning tool. As we mentioned earlier in this chapter, aerobic exercise is responsible for strengthening so many of the body's systems and for diminishing the potential for a long list of life-threatening illnesses. You don't want to miss out on any of these benefits.

Don't become a one-dimensional fitness person. Too many people without weight issues concentrate their fitness program on weight training to sculpt their body. They feel that since they don't have weight to lose, they don't need to bother with aerobic activity. This could not be further from the truth. The heart needs to be worked just as hard as every other muscle in the body to keep it in tip-top shape. After all, what good are large biceps when your heart stops beating?

Make your fitness partnership last a lifetime and keep your heart healthy with aerobic exercise.

No Buts About It

Excuses, excuses. Aerobic exercise is essential to your fitness program and we know with the right amount of encouragement, you will overcome your aerobiphobia and emerge as an aerobic star. You just need to know your comfort zone and your limits, and then push slightly past them so you can learn new skills and reach a higher level of fitness.

Remember, part of your fitness learning process is learning to let go of old ideas and preconceived notions about exercise. So abandon the Jane Fonda and Richard Simmons mental pictures and instead imagine yourself as an aerobic king or queen—fit, healthy, and full of life.

The Least You Need to Know

- Every person, no matter what their current fitness level, can benefit from challenging aerobic activity.
- There are countless types of aerobic exercises that partners can do together.
- Aerobic activity not only shapes the outside of the body, but the inside as well.
- It's important to overcome your fear of treadmills and other gym machines or you will rob yourself of great exercise tools.

In This Chapter

◆ Defining the FITT principle and how it will help you organize your workout

◆ Methods for measuring your exercise intensity

◆ When to vary your routine and when to stick to the plan

◆ Common injuries associated with cardio exercise

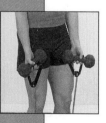
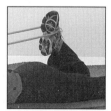
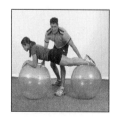
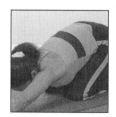
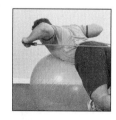
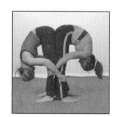

Chapter 7

Cardio Confusion

When it comes to your workout, don't let any confusion get in the way of a great exercise session. We've been talking a great deal about how to get started with an exercise program. Now it's time to show you that all of this is really simple and easy. There's no need for any confusion (but if you do get confused, don't forget that we're here to help).

In these pages, we'll show you how to organize your cardio exercise session including how long, how hard, and how often you should be working. We'll also teach you how to measure your own and your partner's exercise intensity, as well as when to kick it up and when to turn it down. After you read this chapter, you will have a better idea of how you should feel after every cardio workout.

Choose Your Workout (FITT)

There is a simple fitness principle that is the basis for designing all types of exercise programs. It is the FITT principle—Frequency, Intensity, Time, Type. When creating your fitness goals, remember to include the FITT principle for you and your partner in your workout journals.

Frequency

Frequency is the number of times per week that you plan to exercise.

Intensity

Intensity is how hard you plan to work out during each session. The best way to gauge your intensity is to follow the Target Heart Rate Zone, which we will explain later in this chapter.

Time

Time is how long you plan to exercise for each session. One of the things to remember is that the minutes you exercise in a day do not need to be consecutive. Studies have shown that three smaller workouts of 10 minutes per day can be just as beneficial as one 30-minute workout.

You can plan how much you exercise by considering your intensity and the time. Two great choices are:

◆ Moderate intensity activity for 30 minutes per day, a minimum of five days per week or more. Moderate activity is equal to something like a brisk walk.

◆ Vigorous exercise for 20 minutes per day, a minimum of three days per week or more. A vigorous intensity activity is one that puts you at 70 percent of your maximum heart rate.

Type

Type is what you are going to do in your exercise session. This can be activities like cardio, strength, or flexibility. You can also break the type into more detail to include the cardio you plan to do, from biking, to hiking, to swimming, to taking a class.

To get the most out of your cardio workout, first start with some simple stretching. These stretches can include the specific stretches of those muscles that you will use in your workout, can be stretches for those trouble areas that always seem to nag you during your workout, or the stretch can be the cardio activity itself at a much lower intensity.

Cardio fitness activities include, but are not limited to, the following:

◆ **Walking**—on a treadmill or outside

◆ **Biking**—either along your favorite outdoor trail or indoor stationary biking

◆ **Swimming and other water sports**—take the plunge and swim those laps or run in a buoyant vest. Water activities are great workouts that decrease the wear and tear on your legs because of the low impact nature of the water itself.

◆ **Aerobic classes**—either as a group activity at the fitness center or by using one of the many popular video tapes

Don't Sweat It

The U.S. Federal Government spends approximately 92 percent of all health-care dollars on treating disease, and only 8 percent on prevention.

◆ **Sports**—basketball, football, even golf (walking) can provide a cardio workout

◆ **Dancing**—from ballroom to square, getting out there and cutting the rug all provide cardiovascular benefits

The 1996 Surgeon General's report on physical fitness follows the FITT principle. It states that American adults should exercise at least 30 minutes per day, at least 5 days per week, at an intensity of 50–75 percent of a person's target heart rate zone.

Am I Working Hard Enough?

You've made the decision to work out. You're in the middle of your workout, huffing and puffing, and you wonder how you're doing. Are you working hard enough? Are you taking it too easy on yourself? If only there were a way to monitor your intensity level! Guess what? You're in luck—there are a few different methods you can use to gauge your workout intensity.

Working hard enough is important to monitor while you exercise. It is the Intensity in the FITT principle that we just discussed. Getting out and moving is a start in the right direction, no matter how little it may seem. To get the best results out of your hard work during exercise, you should monitor your exercise intensity on a regular basis during the activity. This will insure that you are working out in your optimal workout zone, thus getting the most out of your workout. If your intensity is too high, this may increase your chance for injury and might cause you to burn out. If you are not working hard enough, you might become frustrated when you don't see the results that you expect.

As you progress in your aerobic fitness, there are a few different ways you can measure the intensity of your workout.

Target Heart Rate

The Target Heart Rate method is one of the most accurate of the intensity measurements and can be the most personal and repeatable. As you exercise, your heart beats faster to meet your body's demand for more oxygen and blood by your muscles. The higher the exercise intensity, the higher the heart rate. Therefore, monitoring your heart rate is a great way to monitor your exercise intensity.

To use the Target Heart Rate method, you must first determine your Maximum Heart Rate. The formula for this is easy—it's 220 minus your age. The 220 is a measurement of heart rate (beats) per minute. Ever notice that the heart rate of an infant is much faster than an adult's? That is because every year of your life, you "lose" some of your 91 heartbeats per minute.

So let's assume that you are 45 years old. Your maximum target heart rate would be 220–45 (your age) or 175 beats per minute. Don't fret, it is very unlikely that you would ever want or need to exercise at your maximum heart rate— that's why we use a target heart rate zone.

The target heart rate zone most common is 50–75 percent of your maximum heart rate. You get the most aerobic benefit when you exercise in this zone. Take your maximum heart rate and

then apply both 50 and 75 percent to determine the low and the high ranges of your target heart rate zone. In our preceding example, the low range would start at 88 beats per minute, and the high range would end at 131 beats per minute.

How to determine your heart rate while exercising:

1. After your warm-up, take your pulse for ten seconds. You can easily measure your pulse by placing two fingers gently on either your wrist or your neck. Don't use your thumb—it has its own pulse, which can confuse you. With your two fingers, touch gently—by pressing too hard, you might get an inaccurate reading.

2. Count the beats for 10 seconds. Take this number and multiply by six. This is your beats per minute.

3. Adjust your workout intensity accordingly so that your heart rate stays in your target heart rate zone.

You can substitute a 15-second count and then multiply that number by four, but we've found that the 10-second count is easier and quicker to do. For a more immediate measure of your heart rate, you might want to consider purchasing a heart rate monitor. Many models with different features are available, so you are sure to find the one you want.

Remember that your target heart rate is just a tool or a gauge of your workout. If you are a beginning exerciser in a cardio-fitness program, you should aim for the lower end of the intensity zone and gradually pick up the intensity as you become more comfortable with your new program.

If you are a regular exerciser or are training for some sort of competitive event, you may choose to work out at the higher end of the zone. No matter what, remember that each person is different. Pay attention to how you feel—that's the best measurement of all. Keep in mind that the target heart rate zone is recommended for individuals without any health problems. Additionally, individuals taking medication that alter the heart rate should consult their physician for recommended exercise intensity.

Rate of Perceived Exertion Scale

The Rate of Perceived Exertion Scale (RPE) is more of a "how do you feel" kind of scale. The most widely used scale is from zero to ten, zero being very easy, and ten being very difficult. While exercising, either your partner can ask you, or you can ask yourself, to rank your difficulty level between zero and ten. You will want to shoot for a range of three to five for an RPE scale to maximize your aerobic fitness session. For example, sitting silently in a chair would have a rating of zero. Standing and waving your arms gently might increase the perceived intensity to one. Walking at a pace that you feel is moderate might be given a rating of three.

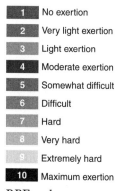

1	No exertion
2	Very light exertion
3	Light exertion
4	Moderate exertion
5	Somewhat difficult
6	Difficult
7	Hard
8	Very hard
9	Extremely hard
10	Maximum exertion

RPE scale.

Remember, the rating of your exertion should be completely independent of the pace you think you are walking; it is dependent solely on the feelings caused by the exertion. If your ranking is too low, raise the intensity level of whatever you are doing. If your ranking is too high, decrease your level of intensity and reassess your ranking in a few minutes. The use of the RPE scale to measure your perceived exertion is helpful in watching your intensity in order to avoid uncomfortable exercise sessions.

Talk Test

The easiest and quickest way to determine if you are working out at the proper intensity, especially with a partner, is to use the talk test. Here's how to do it:

◆ If you can't talk as you exercise, or are completely breathless, you're exercising too hard and should decrease your intensity. Don't try to be a hero—if you feel dizzy or lightheaded, your body is giving you a sign to slow down.

◆ If you can carry on a conversation with your partner with little trouble from the workout, then you are probably exercising in the right zone.

◆ If you can sing your favorite song and do a little dance while exercising, then you probably need to stop taking it too easy and pick up the pace.

One of the hardest things to do when creating a cardio-fitness program is to balance both the intensity and the duration of your workout. There are different schools of thought on whether you should have a workout that is shorter in duration but higher in intensity versus a longer duration and a lower intensity. Here are some guidelines:

◆ If you are a beginning exerciser, you might want to consider a workout that is lower in intensity and longer in duration. The last thing you want to do is to create an environment that would cause you not to work out. Many times, beginning exercisers are eager to begin and overdo their first few workouts.

◆ If you find your daily life to be busy, you might consider a higher intensity and a shorter duration. A quick 30-minute run, or a step machine on a higher level, will allow you to burn those calories and really give you a great workout.

◆ If you are recovering from an injury, you might want to consider a lower intensity and a longer duration. This will help you feel good about doing at least something during your injury, even if it is not at the intensity you would have liked.

◆ If you are training for a sport-specific activity like a short running race or a swim meet, you will want to train just like your event, hard and fast.

How Long Before I Change My Routine?

If you are a beginning exerciser, plan to stick with the same exercise program for at least 21 days. Studies show that if you can sustain any activity for at least 21 days, the activity will become a habit, and once a habit, you are more likely to sustain the activity. Once you have created the habit of exercise, there might be a number of different reasons why you would want to change your workout routine.

One of the main culprits is boredom—if you begin to hate the thought of your workout and while doing it, can't wait until it is done, this is a strong sign that it's time to change your workout. One great way to minimize your workout boredom is to cross-train, meaning take the total amount of time that you plan to exercise and split the time into different activities. For example, if you plan to exercise for a total of 45 minutes, you can start off with a vigorous 15-minute stationary bike ride, followed by 15 minutes of the elliptical machine, and finish with a 15-minute run. Think of it as your own little workout triathlon.

Another signal that it's time to change your workout routine is when you feel that you have reached a plateau. As you progress along your fitness journey, your body will "learn" the stresses and intensities that you place upon it. When this happens, and you feel that you just aren't getting the same intensity from your workout as you did a few weeks ago, it's time

to make some minor adjustments and tweak your workout.

You can do a number of different things to change your workout. Think back to the FITT principle (Frequency, Intensity, Time, and Type). You can change the number of workouts per week, or you can change the intensity by increasing your target heart-rate zone, or change the workout time. You will notice that a change in one of the factors will also allow you to make changes in the others. For example:

◆ If you have been working out cardio style three days a week for 60 minutes per session, consider making a change to five days a week and 45 minutes per session. The reverse holds true as well—decrease the frequency and increase the time if "life" and "work" get in the way.

◆ If your partner is on business travel at the end of the week, consider changing your Monday, Wednesday, Friday cardio workouts to Monday, Tuesday, Wednesday. Having your partner for that extra day will go a long way toward meeting your goals.

◆ Don't feel as though you and your partner need to exercise on the same day, the same way, and at the same time for the workout to be effective. Minor changes will actually help your overall fitness goal by decreasing overuse injuries and decreasing any boredom or lack of motivation.

◆ Go back to your fitness journal and plan some different cardio workouts for you and your partner. Getting ready for summer? Then make May your outdoor running month. Ski season fast approaching? Then make November your stair-climbing month.

◆ As in any relationship, be considerate of your partner's wants and needs. Chances are that their likes don't exactly match your likes. You may like outdoor running, but your partner might rather run on the treadmill or even swim. Keep an open line of communication and all will be well.

Daily Activities for Aerobic Fitness

You don't need expensive equipment at home or regular visits to your local gym to get a taste of aerobic fitness. Our forefathers got their exercise by the grind of daily life, and so can you. In fact, there are lots of things you can do every day that will add little spurts of cardio fitness—and you won't even know you're exercising!

- Next time at the mall or grocery store, consider parking further away from the store and walking the extra distance as a mini-workout.

- Did you know that gardening is considered a cardiovascular activity? To add some extra exercise to your garden workout, pull out the old tools our forefathers used—like a push mower, hand trimmers or an axe—rather than the electric version.

- Live in a northern climate that gets lots of snow? Ditch the snow blower and pull out the old reliable snow shovel—a great wintertime workout!

- Man's best friend can also be a great workout buddy. Taking Fido on his daily walk not only gets you out of the house and moving, but does wonders for Fido's midsection, too!

- Instead of driving for short trips, consider walking. Walking not only helps with your cardio fitness, but it also helps strengthen your bones because walking is a weight-bearing exercise.

- Even cleaning the house can be a cardio fitness event. Find some music you like with a quick beat, and try to clean to the beat, thus increasing your heart rate. Don't forget to cool down!

Workplace Activities for Aerobic Fitness

Think about it, you spend most of your waking day at your office, so why not take advantage of that fact and exercise at work? It isn't as hard as you think it might be.

- You may be lucky enough to work at a company that sees the value of fitness and wellness and might offer an onsite fitness center for all employees.

- Work on the fourth floor? Why not take the steps rather than the elevator? Or take the elevator half way up and walk the rest of the way. Imagine the number of floors you will climb in the course of a week and how many calories you will burn doing so.

- Why not take a quick walk around the block during your lunch hour? Or actually walk someplace for lunch, eat a healthy and nutritious meal, then walk back to the office? Exercise and good nutrition at lunch, killing two birds with one stone.

- Rather than using the phone to call a co-worker down the hall, get up and move those legs! Take a quick walk to ask the question, and then stop by the water cooler to fill up your water bottle.

Injury Corner

One sure way to end up on the sidelines, if not on the injured reserve, is to push your body too far. We all can remember back to high school days when physical activity was easier—ah, the beauty of youth. Well, guess what? Neither you nor your partner nor I can do what we did then, so let's just forget about it, shall we?

We've all heard of a person collapsing and dying of a heart attack while running a 5K. Thankfully, this is a rare occurrence. These athletes typically had some sort of underlying problem that combined with the exercise to cause their death. That is why every credible fitness professional or book will suggest that if you have any sort of medical problem or think you might have a problem, you should visit your doctor before beginning your workout. Better safe than sorry.

The most common injury risk associated with physical activity is an injury that occurs during the activity itself to the musculoskeletal system— the muscles, bones, joints, or tendons. With a little preplanning and listening to your body, you and your partner can avoid these nagging injuries. In most cases, the injuries are usually not serious and often require no treatment other than a few days of rest. If you haven't run more than a few miles and you decide to get out and go gung-ho by running ten miles, you can be assured of some sort of pain the next day. Just use your common sense and build up to the desired level gradually.

So what can you do to reduce your chances for injury during exercise?

◆ **Use common sense.** If something doesn't feel right, stop and listen to your body. An ache here or a pain there might be your body telling you to slow down before the real pain hits! Remember, this is supposed to be fun.

◆ **Stretch, stretch, stretch.** Stretching before your workout improves joint flexibility and limbers tight muscles, thereby reducing your risk of tears and sprains. Concentrate on stretching those muscle groups used in your particular activity. Stretching for a few minutes after exercise is also recommended to prevent muscle soreness.

◆ **Warm-up and cool down.** Let your body get prepared for whatever activity you plan to tackle. Use your partner as a good gauge for when to increase your activity. After the workout, remember to cool down and slowly bring things back to normal.

◆ **Use the right equipment.** If you haven't run a mile in years but have your old track shoes in the back of your closet, you might want to go out and get a new pair of running shoes. Technology has changed in the years since high school and your partner will also be happy for the two of you not being stopped by the fitness fashion police. Whatever your activity, be sure that your equipment is in top condition prior to use.

The Least You Need to Know

◆ Remember the FITT principle— Frequency, Intensity, Time, and Type.

◆ The "talk test," rate of perceived exertion (RPE), and taking your heart rate are three ways to monitor your aerobic exercise intensity.

◆ You can do hundreds of different at-home and at-work everyday activities to increase the amount of aerobic fitness you get in a day.

◆ Your mission, should you choose to accept it, is to exercise your heart (through aerobic fitness) for 30 minutes per day on most days of the week.

In This Chapter

- ◆ How to start slow and learn to enjoy aerobic activity

- ◆ Precautions that you and your partner can take to avoid "overdoing it"

- ◆ What kinds of equipment will help you get the most from your beginning aerobic workout

- ◆ Sample beginning aerobic workouts for you and your partner

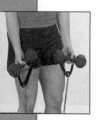
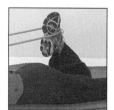
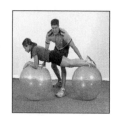
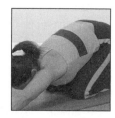
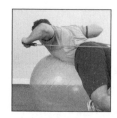
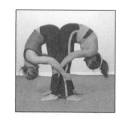

Chapter 8

Work It Out: Beginner

So you think you're ready to start exercising? Well, we think you are, too. This is yet another exciting step in your quest to become fit and healthy. Beginning a cardiovascular workout program is just the introduction that your body needs to your new, healthy lifestyle. The beginning cardio workout that follows lays the foundation for your fitness development. You'll be introducing some major changes in your body, so start slowly and build. Listen to your body and your partner and progress when both are ready.

In this chapter, we'll outline some beginner cardio workouts that will get you started on the right foot. We'll share some ideas for maximizing your workouts whether you are inside or outside the gym. We'll also introduce some equipment that you can purchase to outfit your home gym.

Now start moving!

The Basics

Before you jump in with both feet to your new cardio workout program, we'd like to remind you about the importance of starting slow. Imagine your aging car sitting in your driveway on a cold winter morning. When you go out to start it for the first time in a while, what do you do? You turn the key in the ignition and you let her run for a while. You don't throw it in drive and take off down the street. Doing so would probably be hard on the engine.

The same image can be applied to beginning your cardio workout program. When you jump-start your cardiovascular system for the first time in a long time, you want to let it warm up for a while before you throw it in gear. We know you're anxious to get your heart pumping, but going full throttle from the start will no doubt be hard on your engine.

Fit Facts

To avoid overdoing it on your first few workouts, follow this simple rule: On your first time out, do exactly half of what you think you can do. On your second time, do three-quarters of what you think you can do. On your third time out, go the whole distance. By this point, your body should be used to the idea of exercise and will thank you for the slow introduction.

In addition to starting slow, here are a few more basic tips to help get you started:

- **Start off with a new set of feet.** Well, maybe not a new set of feet, but at least a new pair of shoes. Don't start your workout program wearing the same beat-up sneakers you wear to mow the lawn. Your feet deserve much better. You and your partner should take a field trip to your local shoe store and each invest in a pair of shoes designed for the type of exercise you'll be doing. Enlist the help of the store professional when you make your decision.
- **Try new things.** It's easy to start with something you're comfortable with; we encourage that. But also try to incorporate new activities into your workout sessions. Doing the same thing can lead to boredom and misery and you don't want that to happen when you are just starting out. Introduce a new activity with your partner each week, even if you only do it once.
- **Fuel your body.** Almost immediately, you may notice an increase in your appetite. Your body is burning more calories through exercise, and demanding more to keep it going. Don't ignore your stomach growls. Instead add several small snacks throughout the day to keep your system regulated and your body stocked with energy.

Workout Worries

Some people mistake thirst for hunger. Before you reach for a calorie-rich snack, drink some water. Your body may just be craving the water it lost during your workout.

- **Stretch!** If you haven't been exercising for a while, starting a fitness program is going to cause your body to react, and it may not be happy at first. Expect some muscle soreness and combat it with lots of stretching after each workout. If you are really sore, stretch before and after your workout. Just make sure your muscles are warm before you attempt to stretch. Stretching a cold muscle can lead to injury.

Workout Worries

There is a big debate as to whether you should stretch before a workout or after. The most important thing is that you stretch the muscle when it is warm. If you like to stretch before your workout, start with 5 to 10 minutes of aerobic activity to get the muscles warm, and then stretch. Never stretch a cold muscle, or you will end up with a hurt muscle, too.

◆ **Be patient.** Many people start an exercise program and expect to see changes immediately. You didn't get out of shape overnight, so don't expect to get in shape overnight either. Instead be patient with your body as it adapts to the exercise demands. Don't step on the scale everyday, or flex in front of the mirrors. If you build it, it will come!

There are several other basic things to keep in mind. First, don't worry about speed or pace in the beginning. Instead focus on steadily increasing your endurance. Try to go a little longer or a little further every time. Too many people make the mistake of trying to go fast. Like the turtle says, slow and steady wins the race—or at least finishes with a smile.

Second, don't let your partner's current fitness level slow you down. While you are both probably beginners, one of you may be in better shape than the other. Don't let this minor obstacle throw you off. We'll teach you some tips for keeping an even playing field later in this chapter.

Lastly, enjoy yourself. It's important to begin your exercise adventure with a positive attitude, and keep that positive attitude as you improve. Only engage in activities that you enjoy, or you will likely develop ill feelings about exercise all together. Keep it safe, keep in interesting, and most of all, keep it fun.

Tools of the Trade

For your beginner workout, we're going to keep things simple. No need to invest in big machines or fancy gadgets just yet. Instead use this time to get to know your likes and dislikes. No sense in buying a home treadmill if the impact of walking or running is too much for your knees. We're only going to suggest a few things that you and your partner should have on hand to make your cardio workouts more fun and effective.

◆ **New shoes.** We already mentioned why, but we'll repeat ourselves for clarity. New sneakers are essential for starting out. You want to give your feet the best possible experience during your exercise sessions. Poor footwear will leave them achy and bruised and unwilling to carry you to the next workout.

◆ **A pedometer.** Knowing how far you and your partner walk or run will help you to progress with your beginning cardio workout. *Pedometers* vary in price and quality, so look for something that's not too cheap and not too expensive. Since the pedometer won't be 100 percent accurate, it's best if both you and your partner use one and take the average of the two distances to track how far you've walked or run.

Training Notes

Pedometers are instruments that measure the distance you travel by foot by responding to the body motion at each step. Pedometers usually clip to a belt or waistband of your pants and track the number of steps you take.

◆ **Heart Rate Monitor.** Sometimes the challenge for new exercisers is to determine whether they are working hard enough to achieve results. While any activity is better than none, working within your target heart rate range is the best way to monitor the intensity of your workouts. You can use the information we gave you in Chapter 7 to determine your target heart rate and use the monitor to track your heart rate throughout your workout. Like pedometers, heart rate monitors also vary in price and quality. The most accurate are ones that ask you to input your age and resting heart rate.

The Beginner Cardio Workout

To give you the most effective workout no matter where you are, we've designed two different types of workouts: At Home and At the Gym. Each workout has a 29-minute format and a 59-minute format to accommodate whatever time allows. While all of the exercise programs are designed to do with a partner, you can do them alone if your partner is not available on a particular day.

At Home

The At Home Beginner Cardio workout focuses on activities that require little or no equipment. At this early stage of your exercise endeavor, we do not recommend that you invest in expensive at home equipment like treadmills or stationary cycles. Instead focus on developing your new exercise habit. Once you have made a significant commitment, you can consider purchasing some equipment down the road.

Fitness Walking

Notice we didn't title this workout "Afternoon Stroll." The goal with this workout is to get you and your partner moving at a pace that will challenge your muscles and elevate your heart rate. Be careful not to get distracted by your conversation. You want to keep pushing the pace.

The following box contains the cues for each of the different walking levels. Familiarize yourself with these definitions before you attempt the workout so you can get the most from your exercise session.

In this workout, when the partners take turns in Level 3, the first partner will recover in Level 2 while the second partner "catches up" in Level 3.

Fitness Walking Tips and Cues

Level 1

Level 1 walking is simply your regular walking pace. This is the pace you use when walking through the mall, or on your regular daily errands. The purpose of the Level 1 walking is to warm you up or cool you down. You should practice a regular walking stride and let your arms swing comfortably in opposition to your leg movements.

Level 2

Level 2 walking is an accelerated walking pace. In Level 2 walking, you increase the rate at which you swing your arms, which naturally increases the speed of your leg stride. The majority of your walking workout will be completed in Level 2. This pace should elevate your heart rate and be challenging enough to increase your breathing rate as well.

Level 3

Level 3 walking is a sprint. In Level 3 walking, you should focus on pulling the back leg through to the front rapidly to increase your stride pace. Arms will naturally move faster as well. Level 3 walking is fast, and cannot be maintained for long. Use Level 3 walking intermittently to challenge yourself, but return to Level 2 to recover when you are tired.

Posture

In all three levels, keep these posture safety cues in mind:

◆ Stand tall with your shoulders back and relaxed.

◆ Keep your head in line with your spine and try not to lean forward as you walk.

◆ Swing your arms from front to back and not from side to side. Avoid a "baby-rocking" motion with your arms.

◆ Keep the hips in line with your leg stride. Do not swing the hips from side to side. You want to streamline your motion.

◆ When stepping with the front leg, your foot strike should be from heel to toe.

◆ When stepping off with the back leg, focus on pushing off with the ball of the foot and swinging the leg through to the front.

◆ Do not try to take larger steps to increase your pace. Instead drag the back leg through faster.

◆ Always keep the abdominals engaged by pulling the belly button toward the spine.

The 29-Minute Fitness Walking Workout

Walking Level	Directions	Time
Warm-Up		
Level 1	Both partners	5 minutes
Workout		
Level 2	Both partners	5 minutes
Level 3	Partner #1	1 minute
Level 2	Partner #1	1 minute
Level 3	Partner #2	1 minute
Level 2	Partner #2	1 minute
Level 2	Both partners	5 minutes
Level 3	Partner #1	1 minute
Level 2	Partner #1	1 minute
Level 3	Partner #2	1 minute
Level 2	Partner #2	1 minute
Level 2	Both partners	3 minutes
Cooldown		
Level 1	Both partners	3 minutes

The 59-Minute Fitness Walking Workout

Walking Level	Directions	Time
Warm-Up		
Level 1	Both partners	5 minutes
Workout		
Level 2	Both partners	5 minutes
Level 3	Partner #1	1 minute
Level 2	Partner #1	1 minute
Level 3	Partner #2	1 minute
Level 2	Partner #2	1 minute
Level 2	Both partners	5 minutes
Level 3	Partner #1	2 minutes
Level 2	Partner #1	2 minutes

Walking Level	Directions	Time
Level 3	Partner #2	2 minutes
Level 2	Partner #2	2 minutes
Level 2	Both partners	5 minutes
Level 3	Partner #1	1 minute
Level 2	Partner #1	1 minute
Level 3	Partner #2	1 minute
Level 2	Partner #2	1 minute
Level 2	Both partners	1 minute
Level 2	Both partners	5 minutes
Level 3	Partner #1	2 minutes
Level 2	Partner #1	2 minutes
Level 3	Partner #2	2 minutes
Level 2	Partner #2	2 minutes
Level 2	Both partners	5 minutes
Cooldown		
Level 1	Both partners	4 minutes

To accommodate different fitness levels between partners during this walking workout, consider taking your walk around a track. Walking in a circle eliminates the chance that one partner gets too far ahead of the other, especially during the level 3 phases. If that doesn't work, the faster partner can turn around and walk back toward the slower partner when necessary. In either case, both partners will get a good workout without having to stop and wait for the other.

At the Gym

Different gyms have different equipment, so we've designed this program for the stationary cycles which most gyms have at least a few of. To mix things up, you can do this same workout on an elliptical machine or treadmill. Just adjust the resistance levels to meet your needs.

Cycling

In Chapter 6, we introduced you to Spinning classes. While those are great to add to your cardio workout routine, the cycling program we've outlined here can be done on regular stationary cycles in your gym. Try to get on a bike right next to your partner so you can motivate each other along the way.

Make sure your seat height is adjusted properly so you get almost a full extension of the leg when you are at the bottom of the revolution. If you aren't sure, ask a gym staff member for assistance. When we refer to levels in this workout, they are according to the resistance levels on the bike. All bikes are different, so you can adjust this resistance to meet your current fitness level.

The 29-Minute Cycling Workout

Resistance	RPM	Time
Warm-Up		
Level 1-3	65–80	5 minutes
Workout		
Level 3	70–80	3 minutes
Level 5	75–85	1 minute
Level 3	70–80	3 minutes
Level 7	65–75	1 minute
Level 3	70–80	3 minutes
Level 9	65–75	1 minute
Level 3	70–80	3 minutes
Level 5	75–85	2 minutes
Level 3	70–80	3 minutes
Cooldown		
Level 1	65–80	4 minutes

The 59-Minute Cycling Workout

Resistance	RPM	Time
Warm-Up		
Level 1-3	65–80	5 minutes
Workout		
Level 3	70–80	4 minutes
Level 5	75–85	1 minute
Level 3	70–80	4 minutes
Level 7	65–75	1 minute
Level 3	70–80	4 minutes
Level 9	65–75	1 minute
Level 3	70–80	4 minutes
Level 5	75–85	2 minutes
Level 3	70–80	4 minutes
Level 7	65–75	2 minutes

Resistance	RPM	Time
Level 3	70–80	4 minutes
Level 9	65–75	1 minute
Level 3	70–80	4 minutes
Level 5	75–85	2 minutes
Level 3	70–80	4 minutes
Level 7	65–75	2 minutes
Level 3	70–80	5 minutes
Cooldown		
Level 1	65–80	5 minutes

As we stated earlier, all bikes are different, so the resistance levels may need to be adjusted to accommodate your current fitness level. Instead of focusing on the actual number, focus on the increase in the levels between phases. For example, if your start with a level 5 in your warm-up, increase two levels to a level 7 for your first interval and so on.

The Least You Need to Know

◆ Starting slow and gradually progressing with your aerobic fitness program is the key to a life long fitness habit.

◆ Equipment such as pedometers and heart rate monitors can help you track your progress as you increase your program intensity.

◆ Differences in fitness levels between partners can be accommodated in a beginning cardio program.

◆ Having a longer workout and shorter workout program can help to keep you exercising when you are long or short on time.

In This Chapter

- ◆ How small changes produce big results in your aerobic workout

- ◆ Adjusting to the increased demands on your body with the intermediate cardio workout

- ◆ How to avoid common plateau and boredom problems with your cardio routine

- ◆ Intermediate workouts that work

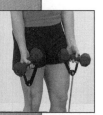 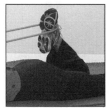 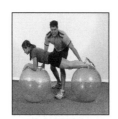 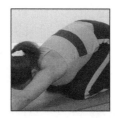 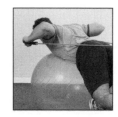 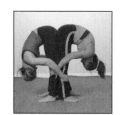

Chapter 9

Work It Out: Intermediate

You're feeling good now, aren't you? You've been working out for a little while and those beginner workouts just aren't challenging you like they used to. You are increasing your endurance, improving your cardiovascular conditioning and generally speaking, getting fitter by the day. This is great news. We think you have finally caught the fitness bug. It's time to step it up a level to the intermediate cardio workout. You want more challenge, so more challenge we will give you!

In this chapter, you'll find more suggestions for ways to intensify your cardio workouts. We also suggest purchasing some additional equipment for your home gym. Once again, nothing too major, just some of the latest toys to build more fun into your workout sessions. Last, you'll receive a few more structured workouts to test with your partner.

Don't waste any time. You're on a roll now. Keep moving!

The Basics

Moving from the beginner cardio workout to the intermediate cardio workout is a lot like taking the training wheels off a bicycle. It sounds like a small change, but it's actually a big jump. While there's a small chance that you'll fall a few times without those training wheels, in the end, you'll be a much better bicycle rider without them.

Don't worry if you experience a few setbacks at first. Maybe you won't be able to make it through the entire intermediate workout the first time you try it. Or maybe you will be sore all over again as your muscles endure the extra challenge. Don't view these as setbacks, though. You're adjusting to the change but your body will be better off for making that step. So take the leap. Your partner will catch you if you fall.

Here's what you can expect as you increase the intensity of your workouts:

◆ **More muscle soreness.** We really hate to break this to you, but muscle soreness doesn't exactly disappear as you get fit. Every time your muscles experience a new challenge, they will respond with soreness. Instead of dreading this muscle soreness, use it as an indication that you had an effective workout.

◆ **Faster heart rate recovery.** Your recovery time decreases as you improve your cardiovascular fitness. Your heart is being conditioned to recover faster and endure more stress without allowing your muscles to fatigue too quickly. You and your partner should notice that you don't get as out of breath as you used to during your workouts, and when you stop working out, it doesn't take as long to bring your heart rate back down to its resting rate.

Fit Facts

To track your heart rate recovery, try this: First take your pulse when you are at rest. The best time to do this is when you first wake up in the morning. Record this number somewhere. Next take your heart rate immediately after you finish exercising. How close is that number to your resting heart rate? Take it after another minute. You should be getting closer to your resting heart rate. Keep track of how long it takes to recover to your resting heart rate. If you have a heart rate monitor, it will actually track your recovery time for you. As you improve your fitness level, you will recover faster.

◆ **Speedier feet.** Were you starting to notice that it was taking you and your partner less time to cover your regular walking route? Isn't that something? You're getting faster! As you continue with the intermediate workouts in this chapter, your speed will continue to improve. Why? Because your conditioning has caused your muscles to recruit more fibers to get the job done. More fibers means more efficient muscles, which means speedier feet.

◆ **More endurance.** Do you remember the days when you or your partner could only do twenty minutes of exercise before getting tired? Now it seems like you could go forever, right? Your endurance will only improve as you get further into the intermediate workout. Now we're challenging you to go harder and go longer and your body is going to respond with a resounding, "Give me more!" Get ready for it.

These are all great things to be experiencing. Your body is finally catching on to the idea that fitness is fun and good for you. Let's keep the momentum moving in the right direction. If we don't, we're likely to hit a plateau.

Ugh! There's that ugly word again. We talked about the dreaded plateau back in Chapter 4 and we're going to bring it up again because now's about the time when you might start to feel the effects of a plateau coming on. You've been working hard for several months, and maybe you've even been losing weight. You're getting stronger, leaner, and more flexible, and you are liking the new you. But maybe the weight loss is starting to taper. That number on the scale isn't going down as fast as it did and you're starting to notice your improvements in your workouts aren't coming as easily as they once did either. Well, then you've officially hit a plateau.

This is not all bad news. After all, you're about to embark on a whole new cardio program, which is sure to break you out of that rut. You'll be trying new activities, increasing the intensity of your workouts and breaking out of the routine habits you were getting into with your beginner workout program. So before that plateau actually hits you, strike back with a more powerful workout plan.

Workout Worries

The first six to twelve weeks of a workout program usually produce the most dramatic results. That's because you went from doing nothing to doing something and your body responds rapidly when you have weight to lose and improvements to make. As you start to improve, it becomes harder to induce the same type of response. It's at this point that you need to increase the intensity of your workout. Your body will think it's starting over again and that's exactly what you want to keep making progress.

Tools of the Trade

Now that you're getting into this workout thing, it's time to beef up your home gym equipment. But before you start testing out treadmills and bicycles, read this section carefully. You see, we're still not convinced that you need to spend a lot of money on equipment to produce the results you want. We keep discouraging the big purchases. The truth is, we're pretty cheap people. While fitness is a big-dollar industry, you don't need to contribute big dollars to make it work for you. Instead pick up some of these cheaper items and we'll put them to work in your Intermediate Cardio Workout.

Jump Rope

You can get a jump rope for around $10.00. You don't need the fancy kind—just a rope with some handles on the end. The jump rope is an excellent cardiovascular tool. And don't worry if you aren't too skilled at the jumping rope thing. We're not asking for Double-Dutch caliber performance. Just the regular turn and hop will work with this program.

Don't Sweat It

Jumping rope was believed to be three times more efficient than any other type of aerobic activity. So the rumor started that three minutes of jumping rope was equal to ten minutes of running. This was based on a study done in the 1960s. However, more sophisticated studies disproved this in later years. The truth is that jumping rope is equal to any other aerobic exercise for cardiovascular fitness.

Stopwatch

Okay, so this isn't a fancy piece of equipment. But if you don't have a stopwatch now, we're recommending you get one. In your beginner workout, we said don't worry about time or speed, just do what you can. Now time is going to become a factor in your workouts. We want you to go harder for longer, and having the stopwatch will help you and your partner keep track of your workouts and the intervals in each.

Medicine Ball

This is not your father's medicine ball! There is a whole new line of medicine balls on the fitness market today. These balls are weighted, and come in several different sizes. They can be used for aerobic activity and strength training as well and are so versatile that we will be using them in most of the "Work It Out" chapters in this book.

Stability Ball

Stability balls are those overinflated rubber balls that are commonly seen in physical therapy setting. They have permeated the fitness equipment market because, like the medicine ball, they are versatile and can be used to perform a complete array of exercises to strengthen the body from head to toe. They are so popular now that they can be found in any sporting goods or multipurpose store.

A Step

Not a stair, a step. You know, that genius invention that took the aerobic class industry by storm in the 1980s? These steps are a great cardiovascular tool, and you don't need the fancy footwork to go along with it. We'll be using them only as a tool to get your heart rate up, so don't worry about learning all the moves. Up, up, down, down is good enough. These steps are relatively inexpensive and can be found in most sporting goods stores.

The Intermediate Cardio Workout

Get ready to step things up a notch. Leave behind your walking shoes and lower level intensity program. We're going to get you moving in a whole new direction and you're going to love the results. Don't be shy. You and your partner need to get out there and be brave. Try these activities that you have never tried before

and learn to love them. Once again, we've included workouts to do when you are at home and when you're at the gym. The twenty-nine and fifty-nine minute versions will help you get a workout no matter how much time you have to squeeze it in. So let's get moving!

At Home

You are going to need a few things for these programs, so drag out that equipment we've been talking about. You're going to need your …

- ◆ Jump Rope
- ◆ Medicine Ball
- ◆ Step
- ◆ Stopwatch
- ◆ Stability Ball

It's best if you can do this workout outside, where you will have plenty of room to spread out. If outside doesn't work, you'll need at least a good deal of floor space to get the most out of this program.

The Workout

This workout format is called a *circuit*. There will be several stations and you and your partner will be moving from station to station at timed intervals. The great thing about circuit workouts is that you aren't in one place long enough to get bored with the activity.

> **Training Notes**
>
> A **circuit** is any workout that involves stations of exercises that participants complete either at their own pace or at timed intervals. Partners will do all stations at the same time.

The 29-Minute Circuit Workout

Exercise	Description	Time
Warm-Up		
Walking	Level 1 fitness walking	5 minutes
Station 1		
Step-Ups	Partner 1 steps up and down on bench alternating lead leg	3 minutes
Jumping rope	Partner 2 jumps rope	3 minutes
Station 2		
Medicine ball*	Partners 1 and 2 toss ball back and forth while shuffling the length of the room	1 minute
Station 3		
Step-Ups	Partner 2 steps up and down on bench alternating lead leg	3 minutes
Jumping rope	Partner 1 jumps rope	3 minutes
Station 4		
Ball Squats*	Partners 1 and 2 back-to-back ball squats	1 minute
Station 5		
Walking	Partners 1 and 2 Level 2 fitness walking	5 minutes
Station 6		
Step-Ups	Partner 1 steps across the bench long ways from side to side	3 minutes
Jumping rope	Partner 2 jumps rope	3 minutes
Station 7		
Medicine Ball	Partners 1 and 2 toss ball back and forth while shuffling the length of the room	1.5 minutes
Ball Squats	Partners 1 and 2 back-to-back ball squats	1.5 minutes
Cooldown		
Walking	Partners 1 and 2 Level 1 fitness walking	5 minutes

For descriptions of medicine ball toss and back-to-back ball squat, see Chapters 13 and 15.

The 59-Minute Circuit Workout

Exercise	Description	Time
Warm-Up		
Walking	Level 1 fitness walking	5 minutes
Station 1		
Step-Ups	Partner 1 steps up and down on bench alternating lead leg	3 minutes
Jumping rope	Partner 2 jumps rope	3 minutes
Station 2		
Medicine ball*	Partners 1 and 2 toss ball back and forth while shuffling the length of the room	1 minute
Station 3		
Walking	Partners 1 and 2 fitness walking	5 minutes
Station 4		
Step-Ups	Partner 2 steps up and down on bench alternating lead leg	3 minutes
Jumping rope	Partner 1 jumps rope	3 minutes
Station 5		
Ball Squats*	Partners 1 and 2 back-to-back ball squats	1 minute
Station 6		
Walking	Partners 1 and 2 Level 2 fitness walking	1 minute
Walking	Partners 1 and 2 Level 3 fitness walking	1 minute
Walking	Partners 1 and 2 Level 2 fitness walking	1 minute
Walking	Partners 1 and 2 Level 3 fitness walking	1 minute
Walking	Partners 1 and 2 Level 2 fitness walking	1 minute
Station 7		
Walking Lunges	Partners 1 and 2 Walking Lunges	1 minute
Station 8		
Step-Ups	Partner 2 steps up and down on bench alternating lead leg	3 minutes
Jumping Rope	Partner 1 jumps rope	3 minutes
Station 9		
Medicine Ball	Partners 1 and 2 toss ball back and forth while shuffling the length of the room	2 minutes

Exercise	Description	Time
Station 10		
Walking	Partners 1 and 2 Level 2 fitness walking	2 minutes
Walking	Partners 1 and 2 Level 3 fitness walking	1 minute
Walking	Partners 1 and 2 Level 2 fitness walking	2 minutes
Walking	Partners 1 and 2 Level 3 fitness walking	1 minute
Walking	Partners 1 and 2 Level 2 fitness walking	2 minutes
Station 11		
Walking Lunges	Partners 1 and 2 Walking Lunges	1 minute
Station 12		
Step-Ups	Partner 1 steps across the bench long ways from side to side	3 minutes
Jumping Rope	Partner 2 jumps rope	3 minutes
Station 13		
Medicine ball	Partners 1 and 2 toss ball back and forth while shuffling the length of the room	1 minute
Station 14		
Walking	Partners 1 and 2 Level 2 fitness walking	2 minutes
Walking	Partners 1 and 2 Level 3 fitness walking	1 minute
Walking	Partners 1 and 2 Level 2 fitness walking	2 minutes
Walking	Partners 1 and 2 Level 3 fitness walking	1 minute
Walking	Partners 1 and 2 Level 2 fitness walking	2 minutes
Station 15		
Walking Lunges	Partners 1 and 2 Walking Lunges	1 minute
Station 16		
Step-Ups	Partner 2 steps across the bench long ways from side to side	3 minutes
Jumping Rope	Partner 1 jumps rope	3 minutes
Station 17		
Medicine Ball	Partners 1 and 2 toss ball back and forth while shuffling the length of the room	1.5 minutes
Ball Squats	Partners 1 and 2	1.5 minutes
Walking Lunges	Partners 1 and 3	1.5 minutes
Cooldown		
Walking	Partners 1 and 2 Level 1 fitness walking	4.5 minutes

For descriptions of medicine ball toss and back-to-back ball squat, see Chapters 13 and 15.

At the Gym

Moving your workout to the gym means having more equipment at your disposal. Take advantage and make use of it all. These two intermediate cardio workouts involve just about every possible piece of cardiovascular equipment that a gym might have to offer.

◆ Treadmill

◆ Stationary bicycle

◆ Elliptical Machine

◆ Stairmaster

◆ Rower

If your gym doesn't have every one, substitute another machine for that station.

The Workout

The 29-Minute Cardio Circuit Routine

Exercise	Description	Time
Warm-Up		
Walking	Partners 1 and 2 walk 3.4–3.8 mph increase incline 1 percent after every minute	5 minutes
Station 1		
Stationary Bike	Partner 1 cycles at 75–85 RPM Level 5–7	3 minutes
Elliptical Machine	Partner 2 strides at 120–150 SPM Level 5–7	3 minutes
Station 2		
Treadmill	Partners 1 and 2 4.0–4.5 mph increase incline 2 percent after each minute	5 minutes
Station 3		
Stairmaster	Partner 1 Level 7–9	1.5 minutes
Rower	Partner 2 30–45 SPM	1.5 minutes
Station 4		
Stairmaster	Partner 2 Level 7–9	1.5 minutes
Rower	Partner 1 30–45 SPM	1.5 minutes
Station 5		
Treadmill	Partners 1 and 2 5.0–5.5 mph increase incline 2 percent after each minute	5 minutes

Exercise	Description	Time
Station 6		
Stationary Bike	Partner 2 cycles at 75–85 RPM Level 5–7	3 minutes
Elliptical Machine	Partner 1 strides at 120–150 SPM Level 5–7	3 minutes
Cooldown		
Treadmill	Partners 1 and 2 3.0–3.5 mph 0 percent incline	5 minutes

The 59-Minute Cardio Interval Program

Exercise	Description	Time
Warm-Up		
Walking	Partners 1 and 2 walk 3.4–3.8 mph increase incline 1 percent after every minute	5 minutes
Station 1		
Stationary Bike	Partner 1 cycles at 75–85 RPM Level 5–7	3 minutes
Elliptical Machine	Partner 2 strides at 120–150 SPM Level 5–7	3 minutes
Station 2		
Treadmill	Partners 1 and 2 4.0–4.5 mph increase incline 2 percent after each minute	5 minutes
Station 3		
Stairmaster	Partner 1 Level 7–9	3 minutes
Rower	Partner 2 30–45 SPM	3 minutes
Station 4		
Treadmill	Partners 1 and 2 5.0–5.5 mph increase incline 2 percent after each minute	5 minutes
Station 5		
Stairmaster	Partner 2 Level 7–9	3 minutes
Rower	Partner 1 30–45 SPM	3 minutes
Station 5		
Treadmill	Partners 1 and 2 5.5–6.0 mph increase incline 2 percent after each minute	5 minutes
Station 6		
Stationary Bike	Partner 2 cycles at 75–85 RPM Level 7–9	3 minutes
Elliptical Machine	Partner 1 strides at 120–150 SPM Level 7–9	3 minutes

continues

The 59-Minute Cardio Interval Program (continued)

Exercise	Description	Time
Station 7		
Treadmill	Partners 1 and 2 5.5–6.0 mph increase incline 2 percent after each minute	5 minutes
Station 8		
Stairmaster	Partner 1 Level 7–9	3 minutes
Rower	Partner 2 30–45 SPM	3 minutes
Station 9		
Treadmill	Partners 1 and 2 5.5–6.0 mph increase incline 2 percent after each minute	5 minutes
Station 10		
Stairmaster	Partner 2 Level 7–9	3 minutes
Rower	Partner 1 30–45 SPM	3 minutes
Station 11		
Treadmill	Partners 1 and 2 6.0–6.5 mph increase incline 2 percent after each minute	6 minutes
Cooldown		
Treadmill	Partners 1 and 2 3.5–4.0 mph 0 percent incline	5 minutes

The Least You Need to Know

◆ When you stop seeing results with your beginner program, it's time to move on to the intermediate workouts.

◆ Anticipate muscle soreness as you intensify your workout program.

◆ You can design challenging at-home cardio workouts with only a few pieces of inexpensive equipment.

◆ Circuit workouts prevent boredom from being on one piece of equipment too long.

In This Chapter

- ◆ How an advanced cardio workout differs from an intermediate
- ◆ How to use your partner to make the most of your advanced workout routine
- ◆ Challenging advanced workouts

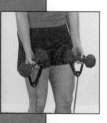
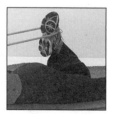
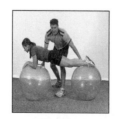
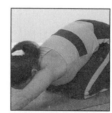
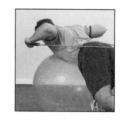
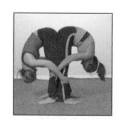

Work It Out: Advanced

Be careful! You've just turned the page to a whole new workout zone. Where the beginner and intermediate workouts were all about keeping you comfortable, the advanced workout is all about pulling you out of your comfort zone. If you really want to take your workouts to the next level, this is the place to start.

In this chapter, we'll be illustrating what a challenging cardio workout really feels like. No more rest. No more recovery. These are all-out, sweat-like-you-mean-it workouts. Don't keep reading if you aren't willing to push beyond your limits and reach your true fitness potential. If that's the case, stop right here and go back to Chapter 8.

But if you're ready to unleash the fitness fanatic inside you, turn the page. Grab your partner and hold on to your hat!

The Basics

Before you start with an advanced cardio workout, it's a good idea to determine if you and your partner are really ready for it. Some people may make the mistake of jumping to this chapter a little too quickly and that could spell disaster for your workout efforts. Of course, you could get injured. Less dramatically, a workout that is too intense could leave you with a bad taste in your mouth. All it takes is one poor workout to kill your motivation and enthusiasm.

So before you make your fitness attempt at the workout routines in this chapter, take this short "Are You Ready?" questionnaire with your partner. If you and your partner can answer yes to at least three of these questions, then you are ready for the advanced cardio workout.

Are You Ready?

	Yes	No
Have you and your partner been involved in a regular cardio exercise program for at least three to six months?		
Have you and your partner successfully finished all of the suggested cardio workouts in Chapter 9?		
Have you and your partner noticed a plateau in your performance and results?		
Have you and your partner determined that your heart rate recovery is less than two minutes? (See Chapter 7 for checking your heart rate recovery.)		
Are you and your partner having trouble elevating your heart rate to your target heart rate zone during your cardio workouts?		

If you and your partner passed our little quiz, congratulations! You should pat each other on the back for all of the progress you've made with your fitness adventure. You should give each other another pat for wanting to take yourselves one step further with this advanced cardio workout.

Now here's the part where we tell you what to expect from your advanced cardio workouts.

◆ **More muscle soreness.** You may even experience more muscle soreness than you did when you first started exercising. That's because this advanced workout is going to be recruiting many more muscle fibers to get the job done. This will translate to great strength gains and improvements, but you'll have to suffer through a bit of the pain first. Just try to remember that saying, "Pain is temporary ... Glory is forever."

◆ **Higher Heart Rate Maximum.** If we haven't made it clear already, this advanced cardio workout is challenging. If you are wearing a heart rate monitor (or checking your heart rate throughout your workout) you may notice that your heart rate climbs higher than it may have with any other workout. Don't be alarmed unless it goes over your heart rate maximum. (Check out Chapter 7 for determining your maximum heart rate.) Exercising in the high end of your target heart range means you will be building endurance to work out longer and harder.

Workout Worries

Exercising near your target heart rate maximum is usually safe for most people, unless you have high blood pressure or related issues. Doctors recommend exercising below your maximum if you have high blood pressure because the increased pressure on the arteries can be a risk.

◆ **Increased appetite.** The reason is pretty simple. This advanced workout will have you burning more calories, so naturally you may feel hungrier during the day as a result. It's always important to fuel your body, but try to avoid bingeing after a workout. You don't want to undo all of your hard work with lots of empty calories.

In addition to these things, no doubt you will notice changes in your body as you adapt to this advanced cardio workout. You may start to notice muscles on your body that you never knew existed! Or maybe you knew they existed but you just haven't seen them since your high school days. In either case, welcome them back with open arms. Your fitness journey just took another turn and this one is taking you straight to the top.

Just remember that every new step takes time. Don't expect to master these workouts, or even be able to finish them, on your first try. Remind your partner to progress slowly and scale back when he or she needs to. You both are there to support each other, and motivation and encouragement are going to be essential to making it through these workouts with a smile.

Tools of the Trade

This is always our favorite section of the chapter. We get to spend your money! But no worries, we're still going low budget here. For your advanced workout, you're going to use all of the equipment we mentioned in the previous two chapters including steps and jump ropes. We're also going to use:

- **BOSU Ball.** A what? A BOSU ball (which stands for Both Sides Up) is an exercise device used to enhance balance and coordination. The BOSU has become very popular in fitness centers because it can be used for many different exercises with many different purposes. A BOSU costs around $125.00, but we promise it will be money well spent. And you'll only need one between you and your partner so you can split the cost. What's more, we'll be using it again in the advanced strength-training workouts, so you'll be getting lots of use out of it.

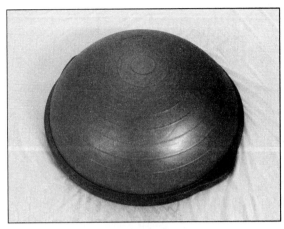

BOSU ball.

- **Treadmill or Elliptical Machine.** This is purely optional. You won't need these for the At Home workouts in this chapter. However, you've demonstrated a commitment to your exercise program and you may want to invest in one of these pieces if you think you have made fitness a life-long goal. While costly, either of these two pieces of exercise equipment can help to add variety to your workouts when you are stuck indoors or tired of the gym. Just shop around and look for quality and price.

We've tried to keep the "Tools of the Trade" list short and inexpensive in every chapter. Don't purchase things that you know you aren't going to use. Nothing is worse than a dusty pile of unused exercise equipment sitting in your basement. No reader of ours will be hanging their laundry on a motionless treadmill, that's for sure!

The Advanced Cardio Workout

We won't talk it up any more than we already have. This advanced cardio workout is a good one!

At Home

Once again, this At Home workout is best done outside, where you have room to spread out. If that's not possible, try to at least set the room up so that you have a few feet of space around each station.

For this workout, you will need:

◆ Jump Rope
◆ Step
◆ BOSU Ball
◆ Stability Ball
◆ Stopwatch

This advanced workout is another circuit workout with stations. The stations are designed so that a high-intensity station is followed by a lower-intensity recovery station. In case you forgot, recovery does not mean rest. The recovery station is simply to allow time for your heart rate to recover to a more manageable exercise rate. It would be best if both you and your partner were exercising at the same intensity at the same time.

The 29-Minute Circuit Workout

Exercise	Description	Time
Warm-Up		
Walking	Level 1 fitness walking	5 minutes
Station 1		
Jumping rope	Partner 1 jumps rope	
BOSU Squats	Partner 2 does squats on the BOSU hopping from side to side	3 minutes
Station 2		
Step-Ups	Partners 1 and 2 step up and down on bench	2 minutes
Station 3		
BOSU Squats	Partner 1 does squats on the BOSU hopping from side to side	3 minutes
Jumping rope	Partner 2 jumps rope	
Station 4		
Step-Ups	Partners 1 and 2 step up and down on bench	2 minutes
Station 5		
Step Runs	Partner 1 runs up and down on step	3 minutes
BOSU Lunges	Partner 2 lunges onto the BOSU alternating legs	

Exercise	Description	Time
Station 6		
Step-Ups	Partners 1 and 2 step up and down on bench	2 minutes
Station 7		
Step Runs	Partner 2 runs up and down on step	3 minutes
BOSU Lunges	Partner 1 lunges onto the BOSU alternating legs	
Station 8		
Step-Ups	Partners 1 and 2 step up and down on bench	2 minutes
Cooldown		
Walking	Partners 1 and 2 Level 1 fitness walking	4 minutes

The 59-Minute Circuit Workout

Exercise	Description	Time
Warm-Up		
Walking	Level 1 fitness walking	5 minutes
Station 1		
Jumping rope	Partner 1 jumps rope	
BOSU Squats	Partner 2 does squats on the BOSU hopping from side to side	3 minutes
Station 2		
Step-Ups	Partners 1 and 2 step up and down on bench	2 minutes
Station 3		
BOSU Squats	Partner 1 does squats on the BOSU hopping from side to side	3 minutes
Jumping rope	Partner 2 jumps rope	
Station 4		
Jogging	Partners 1 and 2 jog or run	6 minutes
Station 5		
Step-Ups	Partners 1 and 2 step up and down on bench	2 minutes
Station 6		
Step Runs	Partner 1 runs up and down on step	3 minutes
BOSU Lunges	Partner 2 lunges onto the BOSU alternating legs	

continues

The 59-Minute Circuit Workout (continued)

Exercise	Description	Time
Station 7		
Step-Ups	Partners 1 and 2 step up and down on bench	2 minutes
Station 8		
Jogging	Partners 1 and 2 jog or run	6 minutes
Station 9		
Step Runs	Partner 2 runs up and down on step	3 minutes
BOSU Lunges	Partner 1 lunges onto the BOSU alternating legs	
Station 10		
Step-Ups	Partners 1 and 2 step up and down on bench	2 minutes
Station 11		
Jogging	Partners 1 and 2 jog or run	6 minutes
Station 12		
Step-Ups	Partners 1 and 2 step up and down on bench	2 minutes
Station 13		
Step Runs	Partner 1 runs up and down on step	3 minutes
BOSU Lunges	Partner 2 lunges onto the BOSU alternating legs	
Station 14		
Step-Ups	Partners 1 and 2 step up and down on bench	2 minutes
Station 15		
Jogging	Partners 1 and 2 jog or run	6 minutes
Cooldown		
Walking	Partners 1 and 2 Level 1 fitness walking	4 minutes

At the Gym

Once again, your "at the gym" workout will give you more equipment options to enhance your workout routine. In this advanced workout, we'll be using much of the same equipment from the intermediate workout in Chapter 9 but we'll be raising the intensity quite a bit. Since you and your partner will be on different machines at different times, you can always choose different intensities to meet your needs. Do what you can at first, and progress as you improve. Here's what you'll need:

- ◆ Treadmill
- ◆ Stationary bicycle
- ◆ Elliptical Machine
- ◆ Stairmaster
- ◆ Rower

The 29-Minute Cardio Circuit Routine

Exercise	Description	Time
Warm-Up		
Treadmill	Partners 1 and 2 walk 4.0–4.4 mph increase 1 percent incline after every minute	4 minutes
Station 1		
Stationary Bike	Partner 1 cycles at 80–90 RPM Level 7–8	3 minutes
Elliptical Machine	Partner 2 strides at 140–170 SPM Level 7–8	3 minutes
Station 2		
Treadmill	Partners 1 and 2 walk 4.2–4.8 increase 2 percent after each minute	3 minutes
Station 3		
Stairmaster	Partner 1 Level 8–10	1.5 minutes
Rower	Partner 2 40–50 SPM	1.5 minutes
Station 4		
Stairmaster	Partner 2 Level 8–10	1.5 minutes
Rower	Partner 1 40–50 SPM	1.5 minutes
Station 5		
Treadmill	Partners 1 and 2 walk 5.3–5.9 mph increase 2 percent after each minute	3 minutes
Station 6		
Stationary Bike	Partner 2 cycles at 80–90 RPM Level 7–8	3 minutes
Elliptical Machine	Partner 1 strides at 140–170 SPM Level 7–8	3 minutes
Cooldown		
Station 7		
Treadmill	Partners 1 and 2 walk 3.0–3.5 mph 0 percent incline	4 minutes

The 59-Minute Cardio Interval Program

Exercise	Description	Time
Warm-Up		
Treadmill	Partners 1 and 2 walk 4.0–4.4 mph increase incline 1 percent after every minute	5 minutes

continues

The 59-Minute Cardio Interval Program (continued)

Exercise	Description	Time
Station 1		
Stationary Bike	Partner 1 cycles at 80–90 RPM Level 8–10	3 minutes
Elliptical Machine	Partner 2 strides at 140–170 SPM Level 5–7	3 minutes
Station 2		
Treadmill	Partners 1 and 2 5.5–6.0 mph increase incline 2 percent after each minute	5 minutes
Station 3		
Stairmaster	Partner 1 Level 8–10	3 minutes
Rower	Partner 2 40–50 SPM	3 minutes
Station 4		
Treadmill	Partners 1 & 2 5.5–6.5 mph increase incline 2 percent after each minute	5 minutes
Station 5		
Stairmaster	Partner 2 Level 8–10	3 minutes
Rower	Partner 1 40–50 SPM	3 minutes
Station 5		
Treadmill	Partners 1 and 2 5.5–6.5 mph increase incline 2 percent after each minute	5 minutes
Station 6		
Stationary Bike	Partner 2 cycles at 80–90 RPM Level 8–10	3 minutes
Elliptical Machine	Partner 1 strides at 140–160 SPM Level 8–10	3 minutes
Station 7		
Treadmill	Partners 1 and 2 5.5–6.5 mph increase incline 2 percent after each minute	5 minutes
Station 8		
Stairmaster	Partner 1 Level 8–10	3 minutes
Rower	Partner 2 40–50 SPM	3 minutes
Station 9		
Treadmill	Partners 1 and 2 5.5–6.5 mph increase incline 2 percent after each minute	5 minutes

Exercise	Description	Time
Station 10		
Stairmaster	Partner 2 Level 8–10	3 minutes
Rower	Partner 1 40–50 SPM	3 minutes
Station 11		
Treadmill	Partners 1 and 2 6.0–6.5 mph increase incline 2 percent after each minute	6 minutes
Cooldown		
Treadmill	Partners 1 and 2 3.5–4.0 mph 0 percent incline	5 minutes

The Least You Need to Know

◆ The 29- and 59-minute "at home" and "at the gym" workouts will challenge your cardiovascular system and improve your endurance.

◆ You and your partner can set the machines for different intensities depending on your fitness level and still get a great workout.

◆ The intensity levels outlined in the chapter are only suggestions. Exercise at a level that you can maintain and are comfortable with.

◆ Substitute exercises or machines when the suggested equipment is not available to you.

In This Part

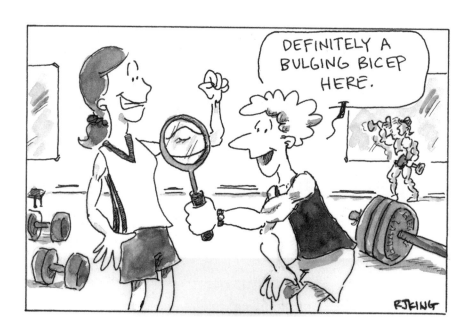

Part 3

Muscle Madness

Strength pilgrimage—the lazy never started and the weak died along the way.

—Unknown

Step two in your journey to fitness is building strength. You and your partner are about to embark on what may actually be the most challenging part of your exercise adventure: lifting heavy things. While you will not be required to move mountains, you will be asked to move dumbbells, which might be just as difficult. It's time for you two to dig deep, summon the strength of giants, and lift each other up.

Strength training is not for the weak of will, it's for the strong of heart. So don't think about how weak you are right now. Think about how strong you are about to become.

In This Chapter

♦ How to organize your workout session to achieve maximum results

♦ How differences in strength can be accommodated with the same program

♦ What are reps and sets and how many should you do?

♦ The difference between muscular strength and muscular endurance and how you can train to improve both

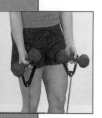
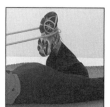
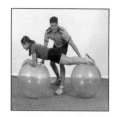
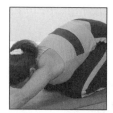
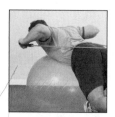
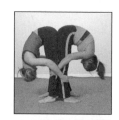

Chapter 11

The Lowdown on Lifting

If you're relatively new to the strength-training world, we realize it can be confusing. After all, it's not like aerobic activity where you pretty much get out there and do it. With strength training, you have to consider reps, sets, intervals, pushers, pullers, assistors, stabilizers … Huh?

If any of those words seem foreign to you, you'll want to read this chapter thoroughly. Here we will define everything you need to know about organizing your strength-training session, from how much to lift to when to take a rest. So read slowly and carefully, and when you're finished, we'll think you and your partner will be ready to move some weight—and not just your own!

Organizing Your Workout Session

So you've got your weights and you're ready to start pumping some iron, right? Before you start throwing your weight around, you need to consider you and your partner's goals with respect to this strength-training program. Are you looking to increase muscle mass or simply sculpt and tone your muscles? Do you want to get bigger or smaller? Also, how much time you can devote to your strength-training program will be a factor in which program works best for you. If you can only strength train two days per week, a total body program might be best. If you can devote four or five days, a split routine will offer you better results.

For you and your partner, the answers to these questions will define the workout program that is best for you. Keep in mind, it's important for you and your partner to have similar goals so that you can both be doing the same program at the same time. Not sure what your goals are? Read through these workout programs and see which best describes you.

Total Body Workout

The *total body workout*, as the name implies, targets all of the major muscle groups in one exercise session. It is most often used for partners who will only be strength-training two times a week at the most. With the total body workout, partners will target each major muscle group with anywhere from two to six different exercises per muscle group. Because the total body workout does work all the muscle groups in one exercise session, it can tend to take longer to complete than some other programs. So if you and partner can spare one hour two times per week for strength training, this is the program for you.

We've used the exercises that we illustrate in Chapter 13 to design an example of a total body workout program that you could do two times per week. For complete descriptions of these exercises, see Chapter 13.

Workout Worries _____

If you are completely new to strength training, it's best to go with the total body workout program, at least for the first few weeks. While it sounds harder to work all of your muscle groups in one session, you'll only be doing it a couple of times a week, which will allow plenty of time for rest and recovery. You want your muscles to actually enjoy the process and not always be sore and tired.

Opposing Muscle Groups

Opposing Muscle Group programs are popular with more seasoned lifters and also those people who plan to devote several days a week to their lifting programs. The concept with opposing muscle group workouts is that partners will be training one set of opposing muscle groups with each exercise session. What do we mean by opposing muscle groups?

Total Body Workout Two Times Per Week

Muscle Group	Exercise
chest	standing chest press with tube
	incline chest press on ball
back	standing back row with tube
	lat pull on ball
shoulders	lateral raise with tube
	shoulder press on stability ball
	front raises with medicine ball
arms	manual resistance bicep curls
	tricep extension with tube
	dips
legs	seated leg extension with tube
	prone hamstring curl
	partner squats holding bar
core	partner sit-up with ball
	tube twist
	side-lying isometric hold on knees

For every muscle group in the body that performs one function, there is another group in the body that performs the opposite function. Take, for example, your arms. The bicep group, on the front side of the arm, is responsible for flexing the arm. On the back side of your arm you have the triceps, which are responsible for extending the arm. Both muscle groups function to move the arm, but in opposite directions. So in an opposing muscle group workout, you and your partner will be training those opposing muscle groups together.

Using the exercises illustrated in Chapter 14, we've outlined a four-day opposing muscle strength-training routine here. Once again, for complete descriptions of the exercises, see Chapter 14.

Pushers and Pullers

Sounds kind of like opposing political parties. One's always pulling and the other is always pushing! Along those lines, pusher/puller workouts are set up so that you work all of your "pulling" muscles in one session and all of your "pushing" muscles in another.

Four-Day Opposing Muscle Strength-Training Routine

Day One

Muscle Group	Exercise
chest	chest press bridge on ball
	push-up clap on knees
	chest press on ball with tube with rotation
back	bent over row with tubing and dumbbells
	back extension medicine ball lift
	lat pull on ball with tube
shoulders	lateral raise side-lying on ball
	stork stance front raise
core	plank with feet on ball

Day Two

Muscle Group	Exercise
biceps	bicep curl with tubing and weights
triceps	stability ball dips
legs	stability ball leg curls
	stability ball adduction
core	rotation with tube on stability ball

Day Three

Repeat Day One

Day Four

Repeat Day Two

To determine which are pushers and which are pullers, just consider the function that the muscle serves. In the case of back and bicep muscles, they are used in pulling motions. Think: Tug of war. For chest and triceps, they do mostly pushing motions. Think: Push-ups. The same rule applies to the legs. Glutes and quadriceps are mostly responsible for pushing while hamstrings are responsible for pulling. If you are paying attention, the pusher/puller workout is the exact opposite of the opposing muscle group's workout.

For this example, we're using the same four-day workout format from the opposing muscle groups. We've just reordered the exercises.

Four-Day Pushing-Pulling Routine

Day One

Muscle Group	Exercise
chest	chest press bridge on stability ball
	push-up clap on knees
	chest press on ball with tube with rotation
triceps	stability ball dips
shoulders	lateral raise side-lying with stability ball
	stork stance front raise
legs	stability ball leg curls
	stability ball adduction
core	rotation with tube on stability ball

Day Two

Muscle Group	Exercise
back	bent over row with tubing and dumbbells
	back extension medicine ball lift
	lat pull on ball with tube
biceps	bicep curl with tubing and weights
legs	back-to-back ball squat
	walking lunges
	step-ups
core	plank with feet on ball

Day Three

Repeat Day One

Day Four

Repeat Day Two

Split Routines

The term *split routine* is used to describe any workout that is not a total body workout. By split routine, we mean that you are splitting the muscle groups and training some on one day and some on another. I know, pretty clever with the nomenclature, right?

Split routines are best for those partners who can devote at least four days to strength training. The reason is this: You want to try to train each muscle group at least two times per week, and by splitting the routine, you'll have to do each workout twice to meet that goal. The good news is that your workout sessions are generally shorter in length because you are only training half of the muscles.

Fit Facts

It's not essential to choose one type of strength-training program and stick with it the whole time. As you progress, your needs will change, and so will the type of program you choose. Don't worry about making the wrong choice, either. All of these strength-training programs will produce results!

Super Setting

Super setting is yet another kind of workout program that can help you to achieve maximum results from your exercise efforts.

A super setting program involves two different exercises and doing them consecutively without rest. For example, you could super set a chest program by doing one set of dumbbell chest presses followed by one set of push-ups to failure. After completing both exercises, you take a short rest break, then repeat the super set.

Super setting is advanced in nature; it is very high intensity, with only short periods of rest in between sets. So we recommend saving the super setting until you reach a more advanced level.

Training Notes

Super setting is a type of strength-training program that involves completing two different exercises consecutively without rest.

Reps and Sets

As if worrying about how much weight you're going to lift wasn't enough, you also have to consider the number of times you're going to lift that weight per set and how many sets you're going to do per exercise session.

Reps, short for *repetitions*, refers to the number of times you are required to lift the weight per exercise. *Sets*, short for nothing, refers to how many times you will perform the exercise during your workout. The number of repetitions is directly related to the goal of your workout program. If you are looking to build size or add muscle mass, you will want to do fewer repetitions and higher weights. If you want to tone and define, you will do more repetitions with lighter weights. When it comes to sets, the same rule applies. If you are looking to add size, multiple sets are recommended. However, keep in mind that the majority of your strength gains come in the first two sets. So overdoing it with sets is not really necessary.

Training Notes

Repetitions refer to the number of times you will lift the weight per exercise. A **set** is defined as the number of successive repetitions completed without resting.

The general recommendations for reps and sets are as follows:

◆ For increasing muscle mass: six to eight repetitions per set; two to four sets

◆ For sculpting and toning: 10 to 12 repetitions per set; 1 to 3 sets

Varying the reps and sets becomes useful if you and your partner have slightly different goals. Let's say your partner is looking to increase muscle mass while you are looking for more sculpting. You both can do the same exercises that we illustrate in the "Work It Out" chapters in this section, only he will be doing lower reps and you will be doing higher. You both can meet your individual goals while supporting each other as well.

Muscular Strength vs. Muscular Endurance

Most people assume that any kind of muscle building leads to increases in strength. When we visualize muscle building, we see muscles getting bigger. However, that is not the case with every type of strength-training program. There are actually several different types of muscle building. We'll take some time to explain them here.

Muscular Strength

Muscular strength is the actual amount of force a muscle can exert against a resistance. To illustrate this, think of Superman lifting a car off the ground. The force required to lift that car one time is measured as muscular strength. Why is this important to you? While we know you won't be lifting cars off the ground as part of your regular workout program, understanding muscular strength will help as you begin to define your strength-training goals.

Training Notes _____
Muscular strength is the maximum amount of force muscles are able to exert against a resistance for one repetition.

When your goal is to increase muscular strength, you are looking to increase the maximum amount of weight you can lift. Workout programs designed to increase muscular strength focus on low repetitions with a high amount of weight because you are trying to increase the amount of weight you can lift every time. You don't care how many times you can lift it, so high repetitions are not important. Muscular strength is also closely associated with building muscle mass, which we discussed earlier in this chapter.

Muscular Endurance

While muscular strength is the amount of force a muscle can exert one time, *muscular endurance* is the ability of the muscle to contract and relax repeatedly. A good illustration of this is Lance Armstrong and the Tour de France. To successfully train for that event, Lance has to train his muscles for endurance, for repeated contraction in order to climb hill after hill. If Lance had only trained for muscular strength, his legs would be strong, no doubt, but they would not sustain him through that grueling endurance event.

Training Notes _____
Muscular endurance is the ability of muscles to contract and relax repeatedly over a long period of time against a resistance.

When your goal is to increase muscular endurance, you are looking to increase the frequency with which you can lift a certain amount of resistance. Workout programs designed to increase muscular endurance focus on a higher number of repetitions because you want to train the muscle to perform against that resistance for a long period of time. If you don't plan on competing in the Tour de France anytime, there are other muscular endurance challenges that may peak your interest, like marathons or triathlons. (But maybe we're getting a little ahead of ourselves here.)

Fit Facts

It is not impossible to train for both muscular strength and muscular endurance at the same time. The best workout program for achieving increases in muscular strength and endurance would be low-repetition super setting.

Rest

Finally! You get to take a break! Actually, we encourage rest with all of our workout programs. Muscles need rest in order to build. Here's why. When you are exercising, the muscle fibers are actually being broken down. It isn't until you rest and allow them to repair that they get stronger. Many people make the mistake of thinking that if they work out more, they will get stronger quicker. This could not be further from the truth. Without rest, the muscle fibers will not be able to repair themselves and increase in strength.

In addition to the actual physiological side effects of rest, giving your muscles a break will keep your mental outlook positive as well. As we have preached throughout this book, in order to make a life-long commitment to exercising, you have to enjoy the exercise. Taking well-deserved days off will ensure that you continue to view exercise in a positive light.

As a rule, muscles generally need around forty-eight hours to recover from an exercise session. Now that does not mean you should only exercise every other day. It only means that you should not train the same muscle groups two days in a row. In the workout programs we illustrated earlier in this chapter, you will notice that you never trained the same muscle group on consecutive days. Instead you alternated muscle groups to allow time for rest and recovery.

Workout Worries

Don't attempt to train the same muscle group two days in a row. Instead allow at least forty-eight hours for recovery and repair of the muscle fibers.

Organizing your weight-training session properly is important to achieving your strength-training goals. However, learning the ins and outs of strength training can be a bit overwhelming. Our recommendation is to refer back to this chapter when you need to, or if you change your goals. Don't try to memorize the different types of strength-training programs that we have illustrated here. That's what you have the book for!

The Least You Need to Know

◆ Not all strength-training programs are created equal, but all are equally effective.

◆ Understanding reps and sets will help you to design a strength-training program to meet your specific goals.

◆ Varying the type of muscle-building program you choose will help prevent boredom in your strength-training routine.

◆ Rest is the most important component of any strength-training routine because it allows the muscles time to recover and rebuild.

In This Chapter

◆ How to maximize your strength-training routine with alternatives

◆ Tips and techniques for being an effective spotter

◆ Strategies for avoiding boredom and keeping your partner motivated

◆ How to pump up using just your partner as the weight

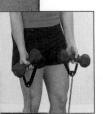 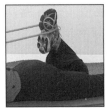 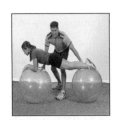 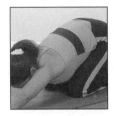 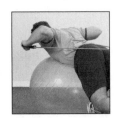 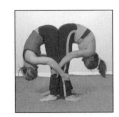

Chapter 12

Pairing Up for Pumping Up

We know you're excited. Those pretty pictures in the next few chapters are just calling your name. You desperately want to skip ahead to see what you've gotten yourself into, to see first hand the torture we've laid out for you. But don't fast forward yet! We have a lot more to cover about pumping up with a partner first.

In this chapter, you learn how to be the best coach for your partner when it comes to strength training. You'll learn techniques for spotting your partner during exercises and creative ways to maximize every exercise for both of you. Most importantly, we'll teach you how to keep your partner motivated when they run out of oomph in their pump!

Overcoming Differences in Strength Between Partners

We spent some time in earlier chapters discussing the importance of finding a partner whose fitness level was similar to your own. However, if you ignored our advice and matched the strength of Rocky Balboa with Pee Wee Herman, fear not! We can help. (Unless, of course, you're Pee Wee and you've just picked a fight with Rocky. You're on your own for that one.)

Overcoming strength differences just takes a little more planning and creative adjusting. Here are some tips to help compensate for the varying strength capacities between you and your partner:

◆ **Steer clear of plate-loaded exercises.** When one partner is much stronger than the other, adding and removing plates between sets for each partner can waste too much time. If possible, stick to dumbbells and machines that can be quickly adjusted.

◆ **Use two exercise stations.** If the exercise requires a bar and plates, like a bench press, consider setting up two benches to use. That way you can move quickly from one to the other without moving the weight around.

◆ **Work opposing muscle groups.** You and your partner can work two different muscle groups simultaneously and eliminate the need to keep changing the weight. For example, one partner can do a back exercise and the other can do a bicep exercise. After you complete the recommended number of sets, switch. This will keep the program moving in the right direction without slowing you down.

◆ **Use your partner as extra weight.** No kidding! If you are the Rocky figure in this scenario, instead of adding extra weight to your exercise, consider adding Pee Wee. This is called Manual Resistance Training, and we'll get more into it later in this chapter.

The Role of the Spotter

Being a spotter is one of the most important roles you will play in your fitness partner career. As the spotter, you are responsible for three things:

◆ Correcting your partner's form

◆ Helping your partner through the "sticking" points

◆ Rescuing your partner if the weight gets too heavy

Training Notes

Spotting an exercise means to safely guide the exerciser through the range of motion.

Correcting Form

Let's begin with correcting form. We're going to get on our soapbox here for a second, so bear with us.

Maintaining proper form during exercise is absolutely essential to success. There are no ifs, ands, or buts about it. Whether you are by yourself or with a partner, you should always strive for excellent form. Every exercise is designed to work the muscle through a specific range of motion. If you slack on the form, you compromise the range of motion and therefore the effectiveness of the exercise. You also increase your risk of injury by about 3,000 percent. While that's not a scientific number, this is no joke. If you don't believe us, believe this: The American College of Sports Medicine says that 90 percent of all exercise-related injuries stem from improper form. Those are odds you just don't want to mess with.

In order to understand a little bit about form, you need to understand *muscle function* as well. When we say function, we refer to the function of the muscle as it moves. For instance, the function of your bicep muscle is to flex and extend the arm and the elbow joint. (Think of raising a glass of water to your mouth to sip.) Therefore, if you were going to perform a bicep exercise, proper form would include flexing the arm while maintaining the stability at the elbow joint. Sounds easy enough, right? But maintaining stability at the elbow joint also means maintaining the stability of every other joint in the body. Why? Because the function of the bicep exercise is to move the arm, not the back, chest, shoulders and hips.

Are you confused yet? Check out the following pictures. The top photo shows improper form for a bicep curl. Note the instability of the major joints in the body. Now look at the bottom picture. Notice how the only joint in motion is the elbow joint.

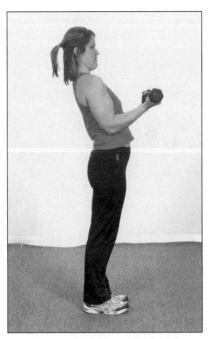

Improper bicep exercise form.

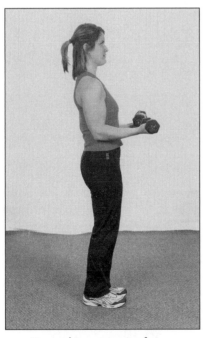

Proper bicep exercise form.

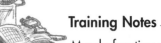

Training Notes _____

Muscle function refers to the specific purpose that the muscle serves during motion.

When it comes to form, your purpose as the spotter is to …

◆ Prevent injury

◆ Maximize the effectiveness of the exercise

The Sticking Points

Okay, now on to the "sticking points." It's easy to spot the sticking point of an exercise. It's usually at an angle just before 90 degrees where the exerciser has difficulty pushing the load over the hump, so to speak. If you're having trouble visualizing, think about rolling a heavy ball up a hill. There is a point at which the angle of the hill can overtake the momentum of the ball, forcing it to roll back down the hill. With enough inertia, or push, you can make that ball overcome that point and continue to the crest of the hill.

As the spotter, you will notice that as your partner fatigues, the angle of the sticking point may increase. At this time, it becomes even more important for you to assist. Don't let your partner quit when the load gets too heavy. Instead, gently assist your partner until they can no longer move the weight on their own. This would be their point of temporary failure.

To spot an exerciser past the "sticking point," remember these two things:

◆ Use only enough force to help the exerciser past the sticking point. Do not lift the weight entirely for them.

◆ Do not let the exerciser get "stuck" or stop entirely before helping. Instead, help to keep the exerciser moving in the positive direction at all times.

Rescuing Your Partner

Last, let's address The Rescue. The Rescue becomes necessary when your partner can no longer lift the weight. Hopefully, this will rarely be necessary because you will not allow your partner to get stuck in the first place. However, on the off-chance you get distracted by Mr. Hot Body at the bench next to you, and fail to notice that your partner is writhing in distress, it may become necessary for you to lift the weight for your partner and secure it on the rack or on the floor. If this emergency situation arises, you need to act quickly, summon the strength of Superman, and remove that weight load from your struggling friend! As the spotter, this is your ultimate responsibility.

Here are some spotting techniques to reduce the risk of injury to either partner during the rescue.

◆ Always position yourself with the highest amount of leverage over the load. In the case of a bench press, it's best to stand on an elevated platform at your partner's head. The elevation will give you more leverage.

◆ Use your largest muscle group to support the load. If your partner is squatting and gets stuck, don't try to lift the weight with your arms. Instead, mimic the exerciser's body position and lift the weight with your legs, as if you were the one performing the exercise.

◆ Encourage your partner to continue to exert himself. Chances are the exerciser can still assist and together you will both be able to secure the weight safely.

◆ Call for help. Don't be afraid to ask for additional assistance. Depending on the angle of the load and the amount of weight, it may simply be too difficult to lift on your own.

Partner Power

Imagine this scenario: You and your partner arrive at your fitness facility to find that it is (pick one) …

◆ a) closed for renovations

◆ b) so crowded that you can't get on any of the weight equipment that you planned on using

◆ c) overrun by aliens who want to use your stealth body to take over the earth.

Whatever the case, you aren't going to get your workout done inside the gym on this day. You've got a bittersweet situation on your hands. You've actually made the effort to go to the gym to work out (which is automatically two points for you) only to find that you won't be able to torture yourself for the next hour. Another score for you because now you go back to bed guilt free. After all, it's not your fault that the gym is closed, crowded, or overtaken by alternative life forms. Guess this means no workout for you today.

Wrong! Desperate times call for desperate measures and you've got to use your resources. In this case, your partner is your resource. You can actually use your partner as the weight for your exercises. It's called *Manual Resistance Training (MRT)*. I know we mentioned Superman earlier, but we're not talking about lifting your partner over your head or anything crazy like that. We're talking about exercises where you use your partner's body weight as the resistance.

If you and your partner fall into that Rocky versus Pee Wee category, you might be feeling a bit nervous right now, but don't worry. MRT can work for all shapes and sizes. Let's take a look at why MRT is an excellent method of strength training.

Training Notes

Manual Resistance Training (MRT) is a method of strength training where partners use their own body weight and gravity to create a resistance load for the other partner.

◆ **It can be done anywhere, without any equipment.** MRT is the perfect strategy to use when you are short on time or just can't make it to the gym.

◆ **Minimizes rest and wasted time.** MRT allows you to vary the resistance of the load without stopping to add plates or change weight sizes. This will cut down on wasted time and allow you to maximize your strength-training session.

◆ **Muscles can be worked to exhaustion safely.** With MRT exercises, the resistance can be adjusted by the spotter as the exerciser starts to fatigue. This allows the exerciser to achieve maximum effort and temporary exhaustion without the risk of falling weights or injury.

◆ **Compensates for differences in strength capacity.** It is extremely effective in the case of partners with varying strength capacities, which is likely your situation.

◆ **Double the workout!** In some cases, MRT exercises are designed so that both partners can be doing work at the same time. Hey, we're all about efficiency!

◆ **Your partner can't ditch you!** You cannot perform most MRT exercises without a partner, so you two are stuck together.

Now we could write a whole book on MRT, showing you all the possible exercises you could do. However our book is on Fitness Partners, so we're going to cut this down to the nuts and bolts. In most cases, MRT involves a tug-of-war kind of principle. That is, both partners work against each other to create resistance for each other.

The following pages demonstrate MRT exercises for every major muscle group. You will notice in the "Work It Out" chapters ahead that we have included some of these exercises in your workout programs. While reviewing these pictures, keep these key MRT principles in mind:

◆ MRT works on the same principles of overload and exhaustion. In order to properly execute an MRT exercise for your partner, you must apply enough force to cause them to fatigue.

◆ Never force your partner to "lock out" their joint while performing an exercise. This could lead to injury.

◆ As your partner begins to fatigue, lessen the amount of pressure to lighten the load. This will allow them to achieve exhaustion.

◆ Emphasize the positive and the negative action of the muscle. Huh? When you are flexing the joint, that is the positive action. When you extend, that is the negative action. So during MRT, you want to keep even pressure while your partner is flexing and extending. This goes for both partners.

Now on to the exercises.

Don't Sweat It

Just because the gym is closed or you don't have any equipment on hand doesn't mean you can ditch the workout for a latte and a Krispy Kreme. Manual Resistance exercises are designed to create the workload of machines without any equipment at all. It's the poor man's workout!

MRT Leg Press

The Manual Resistance Training Leg Press is designed to work the quadriceps and gluteal muscles. As illustrated in this exercise, it is best to use a stability ball between your feet to stabilize your legs and provide a foundation for the spotter to resist against.

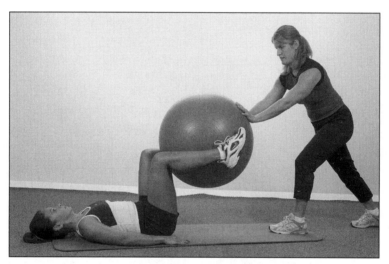

MRT leg press start/finish.

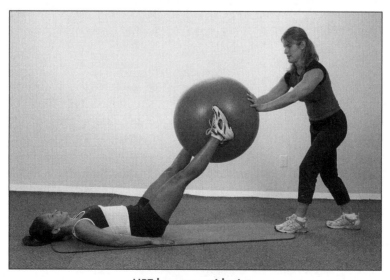

MRT leg press midpoint.

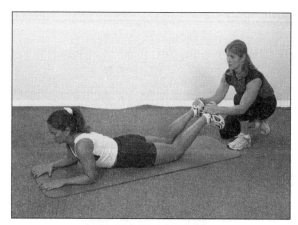

MRT leg curl start/finish.

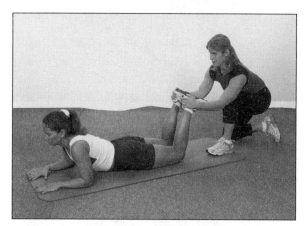

MRT leg curl midpoint.

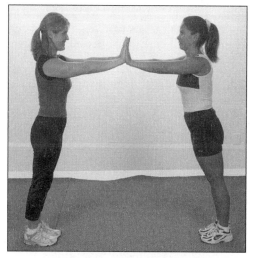

MRT chest press start/finish.

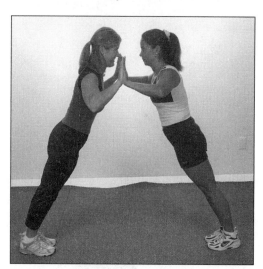

MRT chest press midpoint.

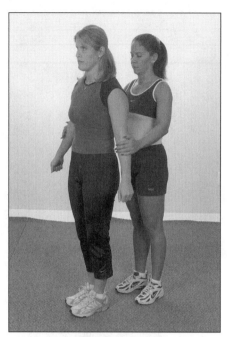

MRT lateral raises start/finish.

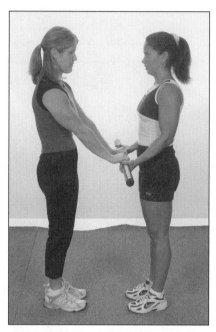

MRT bicep curl start/finish.

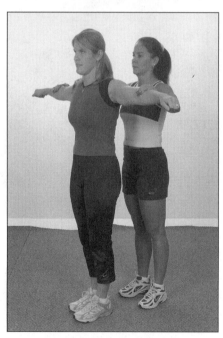

MRT lateral raises midpoint.

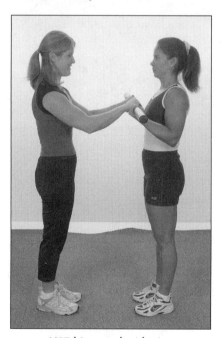

MRT bicep curl midpoint.

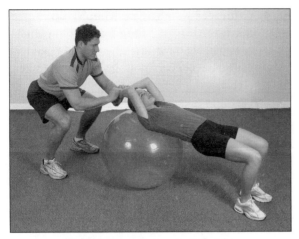

MRT tricep extension start/finish.

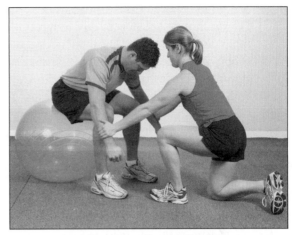

MRT reverse fly start/finish.

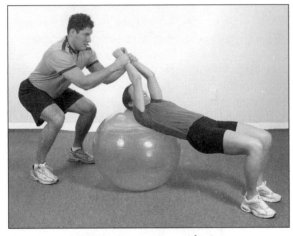

MRT tricep extension midpoint.

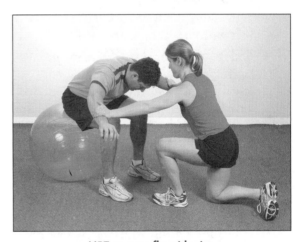

MRT reverse fly midpoint.

There are many, many more MRT exercises that you can do with your partner as you progress; you will see some of them highlighted in the upcoming "Work It Out" chapters. The important thing to remember is that a great workout can take place anytime and anywhere. So no excuses! Got it?

Getting Pumped Up

You're almost to the fun part—the workout! For some of you, accepting that building strength is fun might be a little bit of a stretch

at this point (excuse the pun!), so we're going to share with you some tips for staying motivated. And if your partner is always the one dragging her tail, use these tips to whip her into shape and keep her lifting. If you both can stick with it, we're certain you'll start to see just how fun weight training can be.

We've already spent some time on the basics of partner motivation in Chapter 3, so we're going to cut right to the specifics on encouraging your partner during strength-training exercises.

◆ **Set goals.** Sounds easy enough, right? However, if you're new to strength training, you may not even know what kind of goals you're capable of attaining. Our suggestion is to start by testing your baseline with some basic exercises like push-ups, sit-ups and pull-ups. Find out how many you can actually do before you start your program. Then set a goal that you would like to attain. For instance, "I want to be able to complete ten push-ups without stopping." Then every few weeks, test yourself to see how close you come to attaining your goal. As you increase your strength, you will come closer and closer to success. Need more motivation? Challenge your partner to meet the same goals.

◆ **Chart your progress.** We've mentioned the importance of keeping an exercise journal, and we're going to stress it once again in this chapter. Using a chart like the one here to keep track of the amount of weight you use and the number of repetitions you lift for each exercise will help you to see just how far you've come. We promise you will be amazed at your progress after just a few short weeks.

◆ **Consider a "split routine."** A split routine involves working different muscle groups on different days. For instance, on one day you would work back and biceps only. On the next day, you could work chest and triceps. The next day do a little legs and shoulders. Changing the exercises every day eliminates the chance of boredom and keeps you looking forward to the next strength-training session.

Don't Sweat It

"The best exercise for strengthening the heart is reaching down and lifting people up."

—Ernest Blevins

◆ **Compete in a Strong Man/Woman competition.** We have found that many partners are motivated by a little friendly competition every now and then. Consider setting up a series of strength-training exercises every month to test your improvements and overall ability. For instance, use the bench press and leg press or maybe a push-up and sit-up test. Compete against your partner and don't forget to reward the winner.

Workout Worries

Rocky versus Pee Wee wouldn't be much of a fight to see in the ring, but it can become a great competition around the gym. While your individual goals may be a little bit different, you and your oversized or undersized partner can still set up mini-competitions of strength to keep you motivated. Just keep challenges relative to body weight.

The Least You Need to Know

◆ Partners can overcome differences in strength capabilities by adjusting their workout stations and changing the order of the exercises.

◆ Being an effective spotter is an important role in the success of your partner's weight-training program.

◆ Manual Resistance Training is a great way to get a workout outside of the gym.

◆ Get creative with your motivational tactics. Competition with your partner can really help.

Workout Log

Name: _____   **Date:** _____

Notes:

Exercise	Partner 1 - Set 1	Partner 2 - Set 1	Partner 1 - Set 2	Partner 2 - Set 2	Partner 1 - Set 3	Partner 2 - Set 3
LEGS						
ARMS						
CHEST						
BACK						
CORE						
SHOULDERS						

Basic weight training chart.

In This Chapter

- ◆ Basic tips for maximizing your beginning strength workout

- ◆ Equipment you'll need for your beginning strength workout

- ◆ Pacing your partner for long-term strength training success

- ◆ Total body exercises for the beginner at home or at the gym

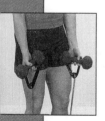
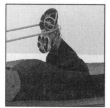
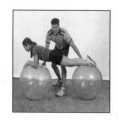
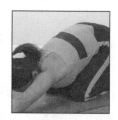
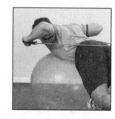
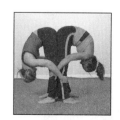

Work It Out: Beginner

Don't be nervous. We understand for some of you this may be your first experience with strength training and that can be a little scary. But you are wise to start in the comfort of your own home (or your partner's). This will help you as you adjust to the challenges of muscle strengthening without being overwhelmed with unnecessary equipment or the distractions that a gym atmosphere can provide. We hope that you and your partner will use this At Home Beginners Workout to begin your strength-training program and then progress to the other programs in the book as you improve.

In this chapter, you learn everything you need to know about strength training with your partner as a beginner. We'll highlight the equipment you'll need to maximize your workout as well as any household items that can come in handy in a pinch. Most importantly, this chapter will provide you with a complete, total body strength-training program that you can do at home. That's head to toe. Nothing left out!

So start turning the pages and see what we have in store for you!

The Basics

If you have never embarked on a strength-training program before, this is definitely where you want to start. This beginner strength-training program is designed to gently "awaken" your sleeping muscles. While they may have been lying dormant for years, your muscles are eager to come out and meet the world and they are ready to start today.

When starting a strength-training program, there a few basic things to keep in mind. Review this list so there are no surprises for those unsuspecting sleepy muscles.

◆ **Slow and steady wins the race.** Do not overdo it on your first few workouts. Remember, you are gently awakening the sleeping muscles, not ripping them from hibernation. If you kill yourself on your first workout, there's a good chance your misery will keep you from coming back for more. Instead push yourself to your limit, but don't jump over the edge.

◆ **A little pain means a lot of work.** Realize that you will be sore after a workout. This is your body's way of letting you know that you worked hard. Muscle soreness a day or two after your workout, called delayed onset muscle soreness (doms), is normal. Expect a fair amount of muscle soreness in the beginning but know that this will taper as your muscles develop.

◆ **Progress slowly but definitely progress.** Continue to challenge yourself as your muscles develop. Just because this is a beginner's workout doesn't mean it has to be easy. If you can do the recommended exercises with ease, increase the weight or the repetitions and continue to challenge the muscles.

Remember also, the beginner workout is not just for brand-new exercisers but also for those partners who have not been participating in a strength-training program for more than a couple of months. If the latter describes you, while you may not define yourself as a beginner, your muscles are starting over and they need a refresher course to become reacquainted with the process of muscle building. However you should not be discouraged. Muscles have memory and once they start to recall the process, your body will respond and you will progress quickly to the intermediate workout.

So whether you are just getting started, or just getting back on track, you are ready for the beginner strength-training workout program.

Tools of the Trade

We hope you read this part before you purchase expensive equipment that will sit in your basement and collect dust. You know who you are. You're the one with a stationary bicycle that doubles as a clothes rack, or an aging treadmill that's great for hanging your ironed shirts on! We know it's hard to resist the late night infomercials, but we beg you: Do not buy what you will not use! And you probably won't use what you buy on QVC.

The items we suggest purchasing are relatively small and can be stored neatly somewhere so they don't overrun your living room. There will be a small initial investment as you stock your home gym, but you will be using these pieces of equipment in all of your workouts, from beginner to advanced.

You can stock your beginner At-Home gym for less than $100. Here's what you'll need:

◆ **Dumbbells.** Since you're just starting out, you don't need to buy a whole set. Start with weights that you can lift comfortably right now, and also purchase the next size up. This gives you a little room to grow.

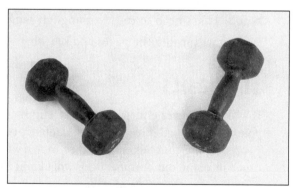

Choose a weight that you can handle comfortably now and then one the next size up.

◆ **Exercise Tube.** Exercise tubes are a great alternative to dumbbells. Unlike dumbbells, they allow you to vary the resistance during the exercise so you can do more before you get too tired. In addition, they are light and easy to pack for when you travel. Exercise tubes come in many different designs and resistances. Look for ones with handles on each end.

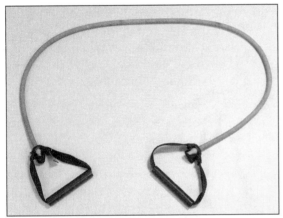

The tube thickness determines the resistance. The thicker the tube, the more difficult the resistance.

◆ **Stability Ball.** They look like a lot of fun, but they're really a lot of work! Stability balls are big, colorful, inflatable balls designed to challenge your core muscles as you exercise. They, too, come in various sizes; however, size does not relate to difficulty. Size only relates to the height of the user. Smaller balls are for shorter people and bigger balls are for taller people. Look for a ball that corresponds to your height. These are usually listed on the box somewhere.

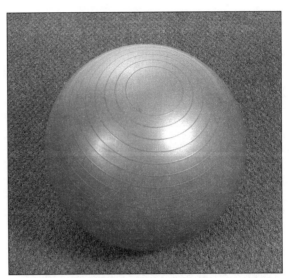

Bigger balls are for taller people and smaller balls are for shorter people.

◆ **Medicine Balls.** Before you get worried, these are not the leather medicine balls of days gone by. There is a brand new breed of colorful medicine balls on the market designed for exercisers just like you. We will be using the balls as another form of resistance, and also as a prop, so choose something challenging that you can progress with.

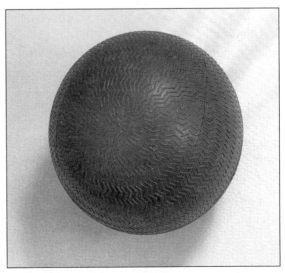

Medicine balls come in different weights and sizes. Choose a size in the middle of the range, probably around 5 pounds.

◆ **Exercise Mats.** While not essential, exercise mats are a great item to have on hand in your home gym. They can provide a comfortable foundation for doing floor exercises and are better than carpet for protecting your back. There are so many different kinds of mats on the market. We suggest looking for one that rolls up and stores easily.

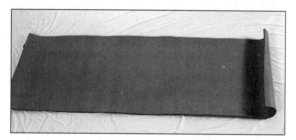

An exercise mat will provide a comfortable foundation for exercises that you do on the floor.

The Beginner Workout

Starting a strength program at home is a little like learning to swim while standing on the pool deck. You really want to jump in and start swimming, but you need to learn all of the safety basics first so you don't drown. When you start an exercise program at home, you are starting with the basics. Don't be fooled into thinking that an at-home workout is not as challenging as one at the gym, though. It just requires a little more creativity and planning.

To get started, all you need is the equipment we have mentioned and some space to work with. Don't worry if the space is not ideal. A little bit of empty floor space will suffice.

Let's get started!

Core

Core exercises are designed to strengthen the muscles that stabilize the spine. These muscles include the abdominals and the muscles along the spine called the *erector spinae*. Core strengthening is critical to overall fitness because it focuses on the muscles that support the most essential part of the body, the spine. While the core muscles are essentially exercised every time we move, they should not be neglected during a regular exercise program.

Training Notes

Erector spinae muscles are the muscles found along the spine that serve to support the vertebral column.

The following exercises can be performed at home to strengthen the core muscles.

Partner Sit-Up with Ball

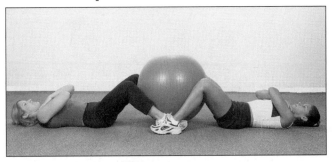

Start/finish.

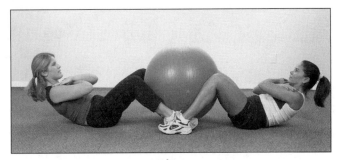

Midpoint.

The primary muscles being trained in this exercise are the rectus abdominis muscles, more commonly referred to as the abs. As you can see, we have placed a ball between the two partners for stability. However, if you don't have a ball, you can simply lock ankles and perform the exercise without it.

Position of Exercisers

Note that both partners exercise during this move.

◆ Partners should sit facing each other with a ball placed between their feet.

◆ Both partners should wrap their feet around the ball for stability.

◆ Begin by lying on the floor with knees bent 90 degrees and arms crossed over your chest.

Movement

◆ Start by drawing your belly button in toward your spine to engage the abdominal muscles.

◆ Keeping your chin off your chest, slowly curl up toward the ball, keeping your feet on the ground.

◆ Sitting tall with chest forward, slowly lower your torso to the floor.

◆ Lower down until the shoulder blades touch the floor.

◆ Reverse the motion and slowly sit back up, bringing your chest toward your knees.

Tube Twist

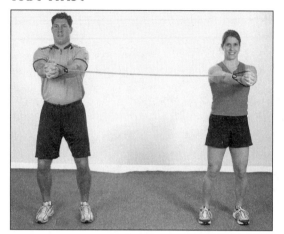

Start/finish.

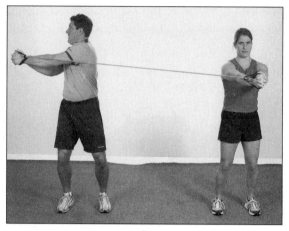

Midpoint.

This tube twist exercise involves not only the rectus abdominis muscles, but the *oblique muscles* on the side of the torso as well. The difficulty of this exercise is determined by the tension on the tube and the distance between the two partners.

Position of Exercisers

◆ Stand with feet shoulder-width apart and arms extended directly in front of you.

◆ Partners should grasp the handles of the exercise tube standing far enough apart to create tension on the tube.

Movement

◆ While one partner stands completely still with arms extended straight out in front of her body, the other partner twists the arms to the outside, keeping the hips forward.

◆ The twisting partner should rotate the shoulders to the outside and then return to the center.

◆ After returning to the center, the partners should switch roles, allowing the twisting partner to remain still while the stationary partner begins the twist.

◆ Once the partners finish one set facing forward, they will turn around and face the opposite direction to work the other side.

Training Notes

Oblique muscles refer to the muscles along the sides of the torso that define the waistline.

Prone Plank on Knees on Ball

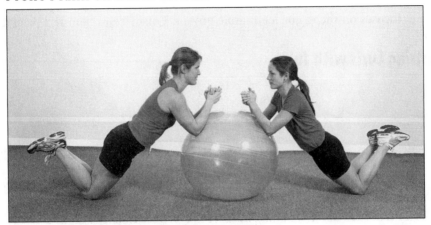

Start/finish.

The plank position is an isometric pose designed to engage the entire core including abdominals and erector spinae muscles. If a ball is not available, partners can modify this exercise by placing their elbows on the floor. Partners should try to hold this position of the exercise for as long as they can without compromising form.

Position of Exercisers

◆ Begin by kneeling on the floor facing your partner, placing the stability ball between you.

◆ Both partners should hinge at the hips, placing their elbows on the ball.

◆ Feet are in the air with heels close to the buttocks.

◆ Avoid "sinking in" to the shoulders by keeping the spine long and the shoulders away from the ears.

Movement

◆ Engage the abdominals by drawing the belly button in toward the spine.

◆ Hold this position while using your core to keep the ball from moving.

Legs

This leg workout focuses on the major leg muscle groups: Quadriceps, hamstrings, and gluteals.

Prone Hamstring Curls with Tube

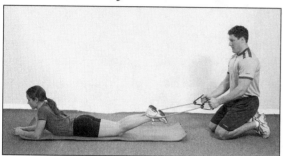

Start/finish.

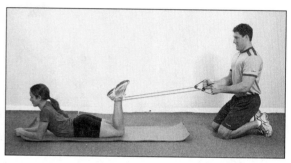

Midpoint.

While the exerciser works the hamstring muscles on the back of the thigh, the spotter gets a great arm workout. If a tube is not available, partners can substitute the manual resistance form of this exercise illustrated in Chapter 12.

Position of Exerciser

◆ Begin by lying prone the floor, propping your upper body up on your elbows.

◆ Bend your knees 90 degrees and flex your feet.

◆ Draw your belly button in toward your spine and contract the hamstring muscles.

Position of Spotter

◆ Kneel about 3 feet behind your partner.

◆ Loop the tube around the ankles of your partner's feet and grab the handles, pulling toward you until there is tension on the tube.

◆ Keep tension on the tube throughout the duration of the exercise.

Movement

◆ Resisting against the tube, keep your feet pulling toward your gluteals as you slowly lower your feet toward the floor.

◆ Keeping the resistance against the tube, raise your feet back up to the starting position.

Seated Leg Extension with Tube

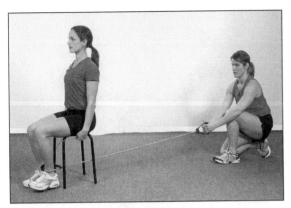

Start/finish.

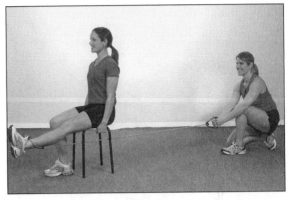

Midpoint.

This seated leg extension exercise works the quadriceps muscle on the front of the thigh. In this exercise, the spotter controls the resistance by creating tension on the tube.

Position of Exerciser

- Sit on the end of a bench or chair and with knees bent 90 degrees.
- Position hands behind your body for support and stabilization.
- Slide one handle of the tube through the other, creating a loop.
- Place loop around one foot, letting it rest just above the ankle.

Position of Spotter

- Kneel behind the chair or bench.
- Grasp the handle of the tube and pull until there is tension on the tube.
- Make sure that the tube stays parallel to the floor.
- As the exerciser lifts, keep resistance on the tube constant.

Movement

- Contract your abdominals to stabilize the back and spine.
- Using the leg with the tube around the ankle, extend the leg straight out, pushing against the resistance of the tube.
- Once the leg is extended straight out and parallel to the floor, lower back to the starting position, keeping resistance against the tube.

Manual Resistance Leg Lifts on Ball

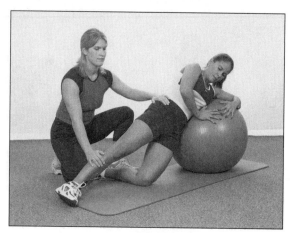

Start/finish.

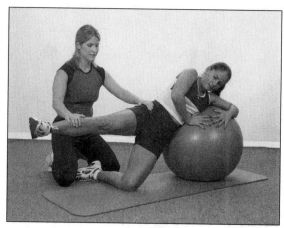

Midpoint.

This exercise combines stabilization of the core with strengthening of the gluteal muscles. The spotting partner controls the resistance by applying pressure to the moving leg of the exerciser. If the exercise becomes too difficult, the spotter should decrease the resistance she places on the exerciser's leg.

Position of Exerciser

◆ Begin by kneeling on the floor with a ball on your left side.

◆ Lean on to the ball, moving yourself into a side-lying position.

◆ Keeping your left knee on the floor, extend your right leg straight out.

Position of Spotter

◆ Kneel behind the exerciser.

◆ Place one hand on your partner's hip to help stabilize her during the exercise.

◆ Place one hand midway between her knee and hip to apply light resistance during the exercise.

Movement

◆ Draw your belly button in toward your spine to maintain your stability as you begin the movement.

◆ Lift your right leg off the floor and continue lifting up until it is slightly higher than your right hip.

◆ As you lower down, returning to the starting position, keep your leg pressing against your partner's hand for resistance.

◆ Lower down until your leg is 6 inches off the floor. Then lift again.

Manual Resistance Leg Press

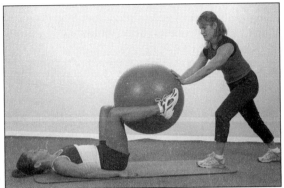

Start/finish.

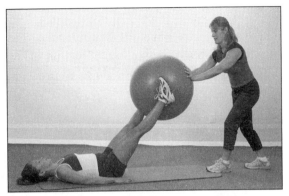

Midpoint.

We introduced this exercise in Chapter 12. This exercise simulates the movement on a leg press machine, but uses a ball and your partner's resistance as the weight. The angle of your legs will also determine how much work your abdominals do, but don't let your legs get too close to the floor or you will lose the effectiveness of the exercise.

Position of Exerciser

◆ Begin by lying on floor with feet in the air, hip-width apart.

◆ Place stability ball between your feet.

◆ Start with knees pulled in toward your chest.

Position of Spotter

◆ Place both hands on the ball with legs in a split stance for stability.

◆ Apply resistance to the ball as the exerciser begins the movement.

Movement

◆ Draw your belly button in toward your spine to maintain spinal alignment.

◆ Press feet out toward your partner until legs are fully extended.

◆ Draw knees back in toward your chest as you return to the starting position.

Chest

Chest exercises for the beginner focus mainly on developing strength in the pectoralis major muscles. These muscles are largely responsible for connecting the shoulder girdle to the sternum, or center of the body. Therefore, any pushing motion of the arms is controlled by the chest muscles.

The following illustrations demonstrate exercises you can do with a partner to develop your chest muscles.

Standing Chest Press with Tube

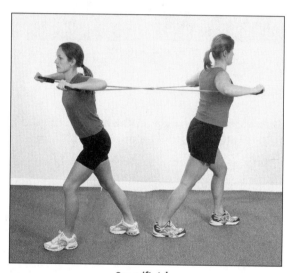

Start/finish.

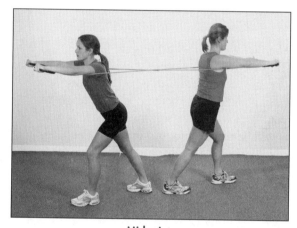

Midpoint.

This standing chest exercise works the muscles of the pectoralis region. The resistance of this exercise will be determined by the tension on the tube and the distance between the two partners. Resistance will increase as both partners push. If this is too difficult, one partner can hold while the other partner moves. Or, partners can decrease the distance between them, which will lighten the tension.

Position of Exercisers

Note that both partners exercise at the same time.

◆ Twist two tubes together, with each partner grasping the handles of a single tube.

◆ Standing back-to-back, partners bend their elbows and position their upper arms so that they are parallel to the floor.

◆ Palms are facing out.

◆ Partners want to stand far enough apart to create light tension on the tube.

Movement

◆ Partners begin by pressing their hands out in front of them.

◆ Push until arms are almost completely extended and hands come together in the front.

◆ Once arms are almost completely extended, both partners return to the starting position.

Incline Chest Press on Ball

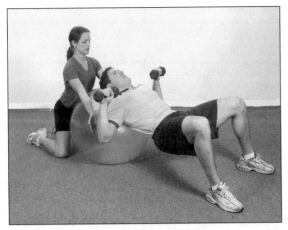

Start/finish.

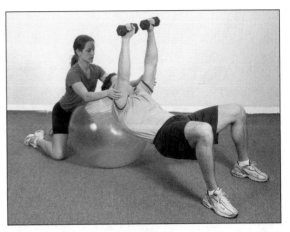

Midpoint.

Another exercise for the chest, this exercise incorporates the muscles of the upper pectoral region. Performing this exercise on the ball challenges the core to stabilize while the chest and triceps are strengthened.

Position of Exerciser

◆ Begin by sitting on the ball with dumbbells in hands.

◆ Slowly roll down until the ball is supporting your torso, between your shoulders and hips.

◆ Lower hips down toward the floor, placing your body in an incline position.

◆ Feet and knees should be facing forward.

◆ Position dumbbells directly over your shoulders with the back of your arms resting on the ball. Elbows are bent.

Position of Spotter

◆ Kneel behind the exerciser, placing your hands near her wrists for support.

Movement

◆ Contract your abdominals to stabilize the spine as you press the dumbbells toward the ceiling.

◆ Extend the arms up without locking the elbows, keeping hands over the chest and not over the head.

◆ Return the arms to the starting position by slowly lowering the elbows back down toward the ball.

Medicine Ball Chest Pass

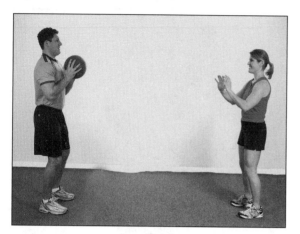

Start/finish.

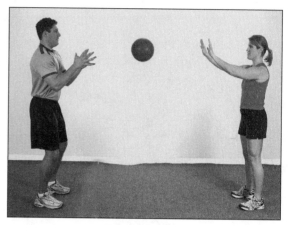

Midpoint.

The medicine ball chest pass is an action-oriented exercise in which partners throw the ball back and forth to each other. During this exercise, the chest muscles, as well as the triceps and shoulders, are working to execute the toss. Partners should stand far enough away from each other to get a strong pass, but close enough so that the ball does not drop on the floor.

Position of Exercisers

Note that both partners exercise at the same time.

◆ Partners begin by facing each other, standing a comfortable distance apart.

◆ Partners stand tall with their feet about hip-width apart.

◆ Partners position themselves with their hands in front of their chests, ready to catch or throw the ball.

◆ One partner begins by holding the ball with both hands.

Movement

◆ Holding the ball at chest height, toss the ball to your partner by pressing your hands directly out away from your body.

◆ The receiving partner catches the ball and draws it in to her body at chest level.

◆ The receiving partner then tosses the ball back to her partner in the same fashion.

◆ Partners continue tossing the ball back and forth to each other.

Back

Strengthening the muscles of the upper and lower back is important for developing and maintaining good posture. Back muscles are often neglected because exercisers spend too much time focused on the front of their body, on areas like the chest and abs. However back muscle function is vital to the mobility of the upper extremities. They serve the opposite role as chest muscles. We've already mentioned that chest muscles facilitate pushing motions. Back muscles, then, are responsible for the pulling motions of the upper body. Each of the illustrated exercises involves a pulling motion.

Standing Back Row with Tube

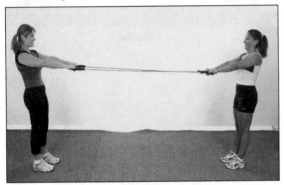

Start/finish.

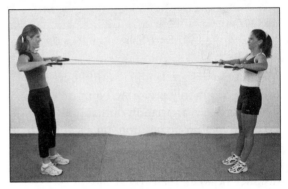

Midpoint.

This exercise is designed to strengthen the upper back and shoulder muscles including the rhomboids and rear deltoids. The resistance is determined by the tension on the tube and the distance between the two partners. Resistance will increase as both partners pull. If this is too difficult, one partner can hold while the other partner pulls. Or partners can decrease the distance between them, which will lighten the tension.

Position of Exercisers

Note that both partners exercise at the same time.

◆ Twist two tubes together, with each partner grasping the handles of a single tube.

◆ Standing facing each other, with arms extended parallel to the floor with palms facing down.

◆ Stand far enough apart so that there is slight tension on the tube.

◆ Knees should be slightly bent and knees and toes should be pointing toward your partner.

Movement

◆ Contract your abdominals and lean slightly back, away from your partner.

◆ Begin to pull the handles toward your shoulders, squeezing your shoulder blades together in the back.

◆ Continue to pull, bending at the elbows, keeping upper arms parallel to the floor.

◆ Return to the starting position by slowly extending from the elbow until arms are straight.

Lat Pull on Ball with Tube

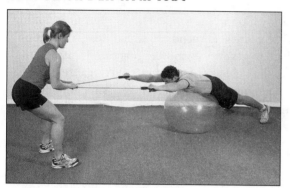

Start/finish.

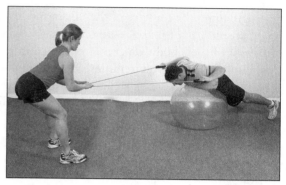

Midpoint.

Most exercisers are familiar with the lat pull exercise commonly performed on machines. This exercise is a variation of that, only it is executed in a prone position, on a stability ball using tubes as resistance. The resistance level will depend on the tension of the tube and the distance between the two partners.

Position of Exercisers

Note that both partners exercise at the same time.

◆ Twist two tubes together, with each partner grasping the handles of a single tube.

◆ Both partners assume a prone position on a stability ball facing each other, head to head.

◆ Partners position themselves far enough apart so that with arms extended, there is slight tension on the tube.

Movement

◆ Begin with arms extended and palms facing the floor.

◆ Partners slowly pull the handles of the tube toward their shoulders, squeezing the shoulders down into the spine as they pull.

◆ After the range of motion is complete, partners slowly extend the arms, returning to the starting position.

Lying Back Extension

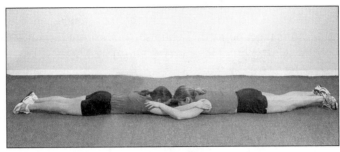

Start/finish.

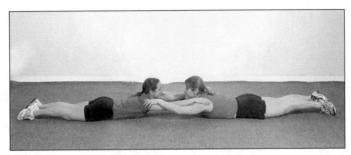

Midpoint.

This back extension exercise is a common exercise for strengthening the erector spinae muscles. Partners should encourage each other to lift as high as they can without placing strain on the lower back. As you improve with the back extension exercise you can add resistance by holding a weight or a medicine ball.

Position of Exercisers

Note that both partners exercise at the same time.

◆ Both partners begin by lying prone on the floor with their arms extending over their heads.

◆ Partners position themselves on the floor so that their hands are touching and their feet are extended away from each other.

◆ Partners keep their heads in line with their spines by keeping their eyes focused on the floor.

Movement

◆ While keeping your feet anchored to the floor, slowly lift your arms and chest off the floor, extending the back.

◆ Partners keep their fingertips touching as they lift.

◆ Once both partners have lifted as high as they can, they slowly lower the chest and arms back to the starting position.

Arms

I don't think we need to explain why arm strength is important. Even sitting at your desk tapping your pencil involves the muscles of the arms. Not that tapping a pencil is necessarily critical to your existence. We're just trying to make a point that you use your arms a lot during your life, and they should look good and work well for you! The exercises illustrated here will focus specifically on the bicep and tricep muscles of the arms.

Manual Resistance Bicep Curls

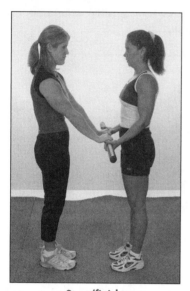

Start/finish.

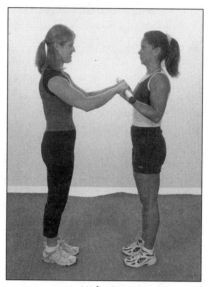

Midpoint.

The manual resistance exercises we described in Chapter 12 can be a great challenge for both partners. If performed properly, this exercise will challenge the bicep muscles of the exerciser and the tricep muscles of the spotter. To increase the resistance, the spotter will exert more force on the bar. The exerciser should attempt to maintain even force on the bar when lifting and lowering.

Position of Exerciser

◆ With palms facing toward the ceiling, hold a stick or bar in your hands.

◆ Bend knees slightly and tuck hips under to maintain a neutral spine.

◆ Keep elbows close to your hips.

Position of Spotter

◆ Stand facing your partner, grabbing the stick or bar with palms facing down.

◆ Apply downward pressure on the bar as your partner tries to lift up.

Movement

◆ Pull abdominals in toward your spine.

◆ Flexing at the elbows, lift bar up to the ceiling, resisting against your spotter's force.

◆ Once elbows are completely flexed, slowly lower bar back down to the starting position.

Hammer Curls with Weights

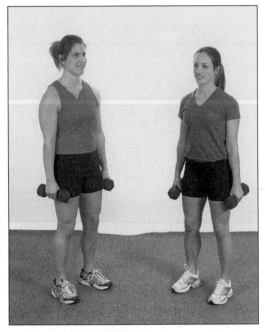

Start/finish.

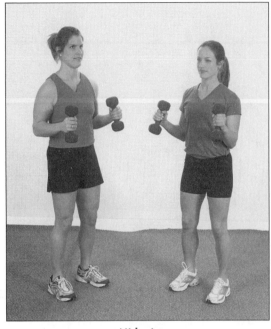

Midpoint.

The hammer curl is a great compliment to any regular bicep curl. The difference between a regular curl and a hammer curl is that with a hammer curl you position the palm facing in toward the body. As you flex and extend the elbow, your wrist is positioned as if you were using a hammer, hence the name. With this wrist position, you can strengthen the bicep muscle at a different angle and fully develop the muscle.

Position of Exercisers

Note that both partners exercise at the same time.

◆ Both partners begin by standing tall with their feet about hip-width apart.

◆ Partners tuck their hips under slightly so that their spines are aligned.

◆ To stabilize the core, draw your belly button in to your spine.

◆ Arms are extended down to your sides, with the palms turned in toward the body and dumbbells in each hand.

Movement

◆ Begin by slowly flexing the elbow and raising the hands up toward the shoulders.

◆ Keep the wrist facing in toward the body as you lift.

◆ Once the elbow is fully flexed and the hand weights are lifted about chest height, slowly extend the arm back down to the starting position.

Tricep Extension with Tube

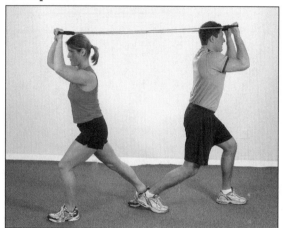

Start/finish.

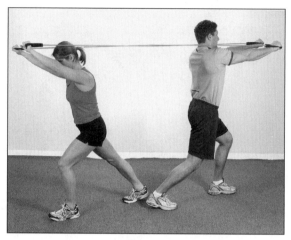

Midpoint.

The tricep muscles along the back of the upper arm are the smallest muscle group targeted in these workout programs. Strengthening the triceps can produce a toned and well-defined looking arm. In this exercise, the resistance will increase as both partners push. If this is too difficult, one partner can hold while the other partner moves. Or partners can decrease the distance between them, which will lighten the tension.

Position of Exercisers

Note that both partners exercise at the same time.

◆ Twist two tubes together, with each partner grasping the handles of a single tube.

◆ Standing back-to-back, partners extend arms over their heads, clasping hands together.

◆ Arms begin with the elbows bent 90 degrees.

◆ Elbows are pointing forward and hands are behind the head.

◆ Partners lean slightly away from each other to maintain spinal alignment.

Movement

◆ Begin by extending the arms, pressing the hands forward to the wall in front of you.

◆ Maintain the elbow position. Do not let them float out to the sides.

◆ Once arms are completely extended, slowly return to the starting position.

Dips

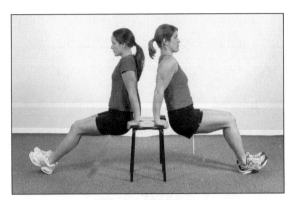

Start/finish.

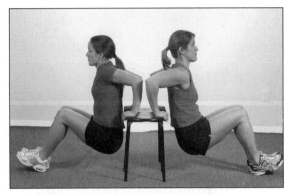

Midpoint.

Dips are another exercise designed to work the tricep muscles. This exercise can be challenging if the arms are not yet strong enough to support your body weight. To begin easy, start with feet planted close to your body. As you progress, you can move the feet further away from the body to increase the load on the arms.

Position of Exercisers

Note that both partners exercise at the same time.

◆ Both partners should sit on the edge of a bench or chair.

◆ Hands are positioned close to the hips with the fingertips pointing down toward the floor.

◆ Knees should be bent with heels pressing comfortably into the floor.

Movement

◆ Both partners begin by lifting their hips off the bench or chair and sliding their hips forward.

◆ Bending at the elbows, partners will lower their hips to the floor.

◆ Partners should focus on dropping hips straight down to the floor and not at an angle.

◆ Once elbows reach a 90-degree angle, partners return to the starting position.

Shoulders

To complete your total body workout, you must finish with some shoulder exercises. The shoulder joint consists of several muscles, the largest being the deltoid group. These muscles are small but pack a big punch. Like chest muscles, shoulders are also involved in the pushing motion of the upper extremity.

Lateral Raise with Tube

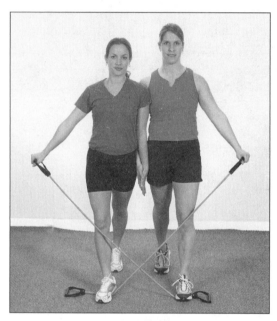

Start/finish.

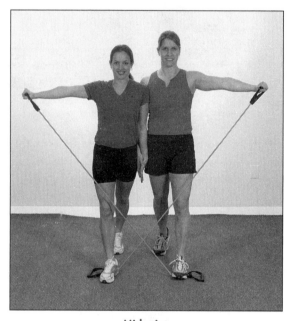

Midpoint.

Lateral raises are designed to work the medial portion of the deltoid, or shoulder muscle. In this exercise, resistance will increase as both partners lift. If this is too difficult, one partner can hold while the other partner moves. Or, partners can decrease the resistance by keeping a bend in their elbows while they lift. If a tube is not available, both partners can perform this exercise using dumbbells.

Position of Exercisers

   Note that both partners exercise at the same time.

◆ Both exercisers begin by standing next to each other.

◆ Partners each grab one handle of the tube with the outside hand.

◆ Both partners step on the middle of the tube with their inside leg.

◆ Partners clasp their inside hands together with arms straight for support.

Movement

◆ Both partners begin by drawing their belly buttons in toward their spine to stabilize their cores.

◆ Begin the exercise by simultaneously raising the outside arm up to the ceiling, keeping the arm straight.

◆ Raise the arm high enough so that it is parallel to the floor and even with the shoulder.

◆ Slowly lower the arm back to the starting position.

Shoulder Press on Stability Ball

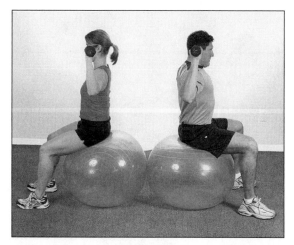

Start/finish.

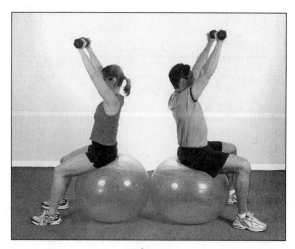

Midpoint.

Shoulder presses strengthen the anterior and medial portions of the deltoid muscles. Performing this exercise on the ball helps to strengthen the core muscles while developing the shoulders. Partners should focus on keeping their spines aligned through the exercise, paying particular attention not to arch the back as they lift.

Position of Exercisers

Note that both partners exercise at the same time.

◆ Both partners begin by sitting back-to-back on stability balls with dumbbells in each hand.

◆ Feet are placed flat on the floor with knees and toes pointing forward.

◆ Hands begin positioned over shoulders with knees bent.

◆ Hips are tilted slightly forward to maintain spinal alignment and prevent arching of the back during the exercise.

Movement

◆ Both partners begin by drawing their belly buttons in toward their spines to stabilize their cores.

◆ Partners press dumbbells to the ceiling, extending from the elbows, keeping hands over the shoulders.

◆ Once arms are completely extended but not locked out, partners slowly lower arms back down to the starting position.

Front Raises with Medicine Ball

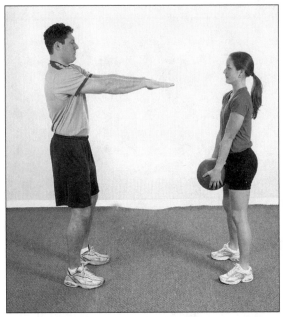

Start/finish.

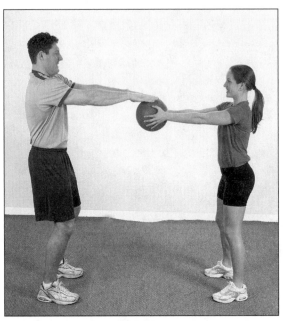

Midpoint.

This exercise is great to save for last when your shoulders are already sufficiently fatigued. Aim for doing high repetitions at a moderate pace. If you do not have a medicine ball available, hold one dumbbell with both hands for the same effect. To increase the challenge, the spotter can continually move the target.

Position of the Exerciser

◆ Exerciser begins by standing, holding a medicine ball with both hands in front of her body.

◆ Hips are tilted slightly forward to maintain spinal alignment and prevent the back from arching during motion.

Position of the Spotter

◆ The spotter stands facing the exerciser.

◆ Arms are extended straight out at shoulder height, creating a target for the exerciser to touch with the ball.

Movement

◆ The exerciser begins by drawing her belly button in toward her spine to maintain core stability.

◆ Slowly raise the ball to your partner's target.

◆ Touch the ball to your partner's hands, and then slowly lower to the starting position.

The Workout Card

The workout card in Appendix B is designed to use with the exercises outlined in the At Home Beginner Workout. Feel free to copy this page for you and your partner.

The Least You Need to Know

◆ The beginner strength-training program is for anyone who is new to strength training or has not been involved in a regular program for several months.

◆ Only a few inexpensive items are needed to stock your home gym, including dumbbells, stability balls, exercise tubes, and mats.

◆ You can choose any combination of the exercises illustrated in each muscle group to get a great total body workout.

In This Chapter

- ◆ The basics of transitioning from a beginner to an intermediate strength-training program

- ◆ Additional equipment you may want to purchase to maximize your intermediate strength-training program

- ◆ Combining beginning and intermediate exercises to create an effectively challenging workout

- ◆ Intermediate exercises for a total body workout

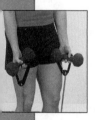
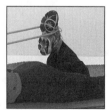
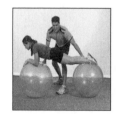
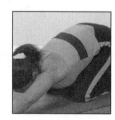
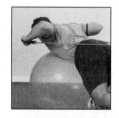
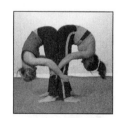

Chapter 14

Work It Out: Intermediate

Congratulations! You have progressed to the intermediate workout. Whether you graduated from the beginner workout in this book or you come to us as an intermediate exerciser, we're glad to be with you at this point. The intermediate workout is a great challenge for your muscles and we know you must be ready.

In this chapter, the strength-training exercises progress to more complex movements. We'll show you how to use the equipment you have already purchased to create new and challenging exercises. We will also be coaching you toward a higher level of muscle fitness as you adapt to some of these new exercises.

So now that you have graduated from beginning fitness, it's time to go play in the big leagues!

The Basics

This intermediate workout is designed for the exerciser who has been involved in a regular beginner strength-training program for several months and has developed enough muscular integrity to progress to the next level. The step to the intermediate level is an exciting one. In this chapter, we combine some of the simple beginner exercises with several compound movements. These *compound exercises* challenge partners to work several muscles at the same time. While some of the exercises may look easy, don't be fooled. Once you start working with some of these exercises, you will see just how challenging they can be.

Training Notes

Compound exercises involve more than one muscle group during an exercise. Most often compound exercises involve a group of muscles that act as stabilizers while another group performs the movement.

Here a few basic tips to keep in mind as you enter the intermediate workout phase:

◆ **Form is power.** Never compromise your form during an exercise to squeeze out that last repetition. Bad form only leads to injury.

◆ **Return to the beginning often.** Again, several of these exercises combine movements. Don't be afraid to return to some beginning moves every now and then. Even though your muscles are more highly trained and you are no longer a beginner by our definition, your muscles still need to remember the baby steps to continue to progress.

◆ **Progress one step at a time.** As you improve, chances are you'll be eager to increase your weights and the number of repetitions you perform. However, we recommend that you only progress one step at a time. That is, either increase your weights or your repetitions, but not both. You don't want to overload the muscle too much or you will be right back at the beginning.

◆ **A little pain means you are still working.** It is true that as your muscles adapt to the exercises, the likelihood of soreness will decrease. However, when you introduce new exercises and challenge those muscles, they will become sore again. That's because you are recruiting more muscle fibers to do the work. Those fibers may not have been involved in that beginning workout, and they are not familiar with the routine. So don't be surprised if you are sore all over again during the first few weeks of your new intermediate workout.

We realize that you might be ready to progress to the next level and your partner may not be. That's okay. The intermediate workout can be performed alongside of the beginning workout that your partner is still doing. Your workouts won't suffer and your partner can continue to progress. So don't ditch your partner. Instead coach him along so he can catch up.

Tools of the Trade

The good news is you'll be using all of the equipment from your beginning workout in the intermediate workout as well. We are only going to make one addition:

◆ **Dumbbells.** You might be ready to increase to a heavier set of dumbbells. In Chapter 13, we recommended you buy two sets of dumbbells; one you were comfortable to start with and a pair you could grow into. If you didn't do that, you probably need that next size up now. If you did do that, you may still want to purchase the next size up after that. If you don't want to do that, you can always combine the two sets you have. For example, if you bought 5- and 10-pound dumbbells, you can put one 5 and one 10 in each hand and now you have 15-pound dumbbells! How's that for simple math?

The Workout

When you start this program, perform the exercises with the same level of resistance that you were using in your beginning workout. So if you were using 5-pound dumbbells before, continue to use them when you go through this workout for the first time. You may quickly move up to the next set of dumbbells, but we want your muscles to adapt to the new activity first.

As you begin this intermediate workout, you may notice that some of the exercises are more difficult than others. We have designed it that way so no matter what level you and your partner are at, you can both have success with this program.

Let's not waste any more time. Get to work!

Core

As your abdominal and low back muscles get stronger, we can add more challenging exercises to continue to strengthen and define your core. Remember, strong abs are not just about looking good in a bathing suit, but about developing good posture and spine health to last your entire life.

Sidelying Isometric Abs on Feet

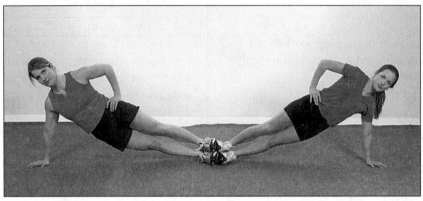

Partners can do this exercise on their knees or on their feet.

Isometric exercises are designed to hold the muscle at a fixed angle. That means there is no movement involved once you assume the position. Isometric abdominal exercises are great for engaging the core and strengthening the muscles around the abdominals and lower back. Partners can start on their knees and progress to their feet as they improve. If only one partner is ready to move to the feet, the other can continue to do the exercise on their knees.

Training Notes

Isometric exercises are exercises where muscles are trained at a fixed angle. With isometric exercises, no movement across a joint takes place. Instead, the subject contracts the muscle and holds the position until the muscle fatigues.

Position of Exercisers

◆ Both partners begin by lying on the floor on their sides with their feet together.

◆ Position your hand under your shoulder and lift yourself up on to your hand and feet.

◆ Keep entire body in a straight line from feet to head.

◆ Be sure to keep hips stacked on top of each other so that the torso doesn't rotate forward.

◆ Extend the top arm straight up to the ceiling.

Movement

◆ Draw your belly button in toward your spine to stabilize the core and activate the core muscles.

◆ Hold!

Incline Crunch on Stability Ball with Medicine Ball Touch

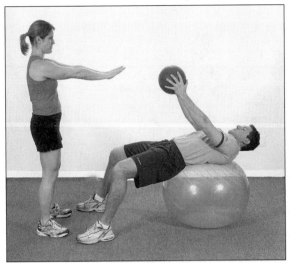

Start/finish.

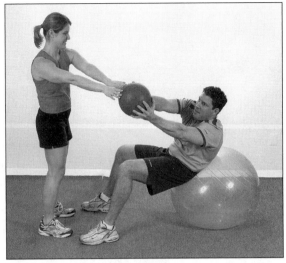

Midpoint.

This is a great dynamic exercise for the rectus abdominis and oblique muscles of the core. In addition, holding the medicine ball will strengthen the muscles of the shoulder during this exercise. If a medicine ball is not available, partners can substitute a dumbbell. For an extra challenge, the spotter can continually move her hand position from side to side, up and down.

Position of Exerciser

◆ The exerciser begins seated on the stability ball with a medicine ball in her hands.

◆ Roll down slowly into a supine position.

◆ Drop hips toward the floor to move into an incline position.

◆ Keep arms extended with medicine ball positioned over your chest to start.

Position of Spotter

◆ The spotter stands in front of the exerciser with her feet directly in front of the exerciser's feet.

◆ The spotter's arms are extended, creating a target for the exerciser to touch with the medicine ball.

Movement

◆ The exerciser begins by drawing her belly button in toward her spine.

◆ With arms extended, slowly curl up into a crunch.

◆ Reach the medicine ball out and touch your partner's hands with the ball.

◆ Slowly lower back down to the starting position.

Medicine Ball Toss on Stability Balls

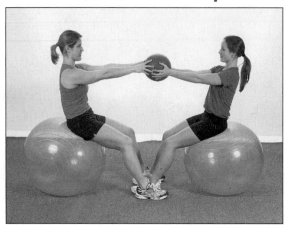

Start/finish.

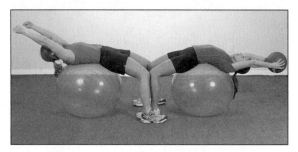

Midpoint.

This exercise is a juggling act! With two stability balls and a medicine ball, this exercise will challenge the core muscles through balance, stabilization, and strength. Partners can lock their feet together in the beginning for extra support. As your abdominal strength and balance improve, you can unlock your feet and give your core the extra challenge.

Position of Exercisers

Note that both partners exercise at the same time.

◆ Partners begin seated on two separate stability balls, facing each other.

◆ Partners can lock their feet together for extra stabilization and support.

◆ One partner begins holding the medicine ball in both hands.

Movement

◆ From the seated position, both partners slowly lower their backs down to the floor.

◆ The partner holding the ball will extend his arms behind his head as he lowers down.

◆ When both partners are fully extended, raise back up to the starting position.

◆ At this point, the partner holding the ball passes it to the other exerciser.

◆ The movement is repeated with the other partner holding the ball.

Legs

You will notice that the leg exercises in this intermediate workout are similar to the ones in the beginning workout with a few major exceptions. Most notably, all of these exercises involve some stabilization of the core muscles. This combination of legs and core is a great challenge for the lower body and torso, paving the way for long, lean abs and legs.

Partner Squats Holding Bar

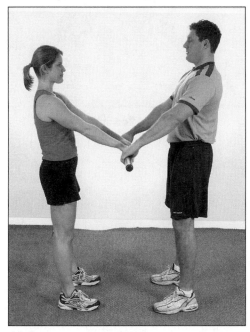

Start/finish.

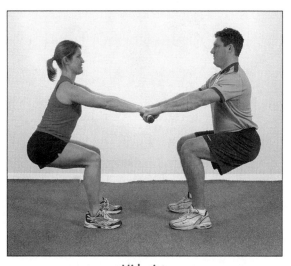

Midpoint.

This squat exercise engages the muscles of the quadriceps and gluteals. Partners may also feel this exercise in their shoulders if the bar is heavy enough. If a bar is not available, partners can substitute by holding on to each other's wrists for support.

Position of Exercisers

Note that both partners exercise at the same time.

- ◆ Partners stand facing each other with arms extended straight out.
- ◆ Both partners grasp the bar with their hands.
- ◆ Feet are hip-width apart and planted evenly on the ground.

Movement

- ◆ Both partners begin to sit their hips back to the floor simultaneously.
- ◆ Keeping chests up and backs long, partners will sit back as if they are sitting in a chair.
- ◆ As partners sit back, they pull on the bar to maintain balance.
- ◆ When knees are bent 90 degrees and quadriceps are parallel to the floor, partners slowly stand back up to the starting position.

Walking Lunges

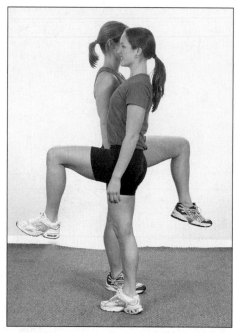

Start/finish.

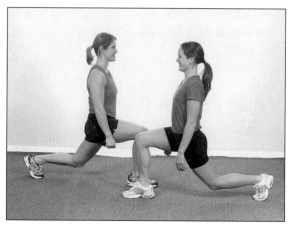

Midpoint.

Similar to squats, lunges are designed to strengthen the muscles of the quadriceps and gluteals. In addition, lunges also challenge the inner thigh muscles, or adductors. Try to find an area where you can take at least ten steps in a row before you have to stop or turn around.

Position of Exercisers

Note that both partners exercise at the same time.

◆ Both partners begin by standing with their feet together and arms at their sides.

Movement

◆ Partners begin by drawing their belly buttons in towards their spines to maintain spinal alignment.

◆ Partners step one leg forward, placing it on the floor and descending slowly, lowering the back knee to the floor.

◆ Make certain that the front knee does not go over the front toe.

◆ Continue descending until the front knee is bent 90 degrees.

◆ Slowly begin to stand up, bringing the back leg through and placing it next to the front leg.

◆ Repeat this movement again, stepping the other leg forward.

Stability Ball Leg Curls

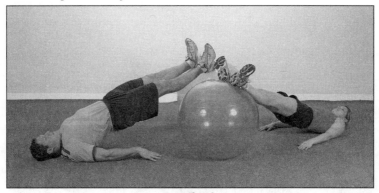

Start/finish.

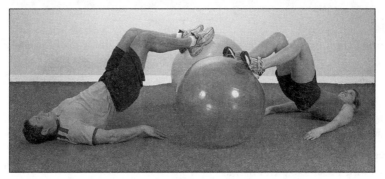

Midpoint.

The primary mover muscle of this exercise is the hamstring found on the back of the thigh. However the abdominals and lower back muscles are also being strengthened while they work to maintain the correct bridge pose for the exercise. For an extra balance challenge, try raising the arms up off the floor.

Position of Exercisers

Note that both partners exercise at the same time.

◆ Both partners begin lying supine on the floor with their feet on a stability ball.

◆ One partner begins with her knees bent and the other partner begins with her legs extended.

◆ With arms resting at their sides, partners lift their hips off the ground and toward the ceiling.

◆ Partners press their heels into the ball to engage the hamstring and gluteal muscles.

Movement

◆ The partner with the bent knees begins by slowly extending her legs, rolling the ball toward the partner with the extended legs.

◆ The partner with the extended legs should respond by drawing her heels into her gluteals, bending the knees.

◆ Partners continue to roll the ball back and forth to each other, keeping hips off the floor.

Stability Ball Adduction

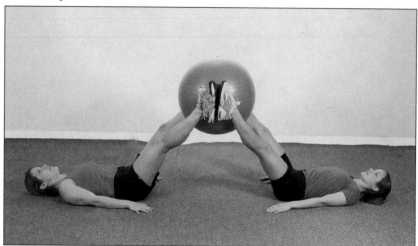

This exercise requires a very small movement from the inner thighs as the feet squeeze the ball.

Targeting the inner thigh, or adductor muscles, can be challenging. This exercise is designed to do just that. In addition to leg strengthening, this exercise also challenges the abdominal muscles to keep the legs stabilized in the air. Both partners should attempt to squeeze the ball as hard as they can before releasing. If keeping the legs in the air is too difficult for one or both partners, this exercise can be performed with the ball on the ground.

Position of Exercisers

Note that both partners exercise at the same time.

◆ Both partners begin by lying on the floor in a straight line with their feet touching.

◆ Place a stability ball between the feet of both partners.

◆ Lift the legs 12–24 inches off the ground.

◆ Draw the belly button in toward the ground to stabilize the spine.

◆ Do not allow the back to arch off the ground.

Movement

◆ With legs in the air, partners slowly squeeze the ball between their feet.

◆ Repeat the squeezing motion until the muscle fatigues.

Chest

With these intermediate chest exercises we focus on incorporating some stabilization into the movement. Don't worry if you can't do everything at first. These moves are complex and will take some getting used to.

Chest Press Bridge on Stability Ball

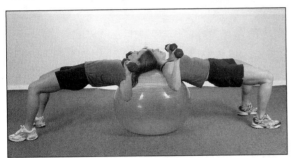

Start/finish.

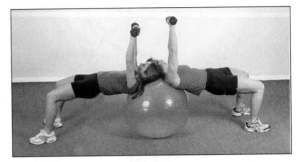

Midpoint.

This multidimensional chest exercise challenges muscles in both the upper and lower extremities. The chest muscles work against the resistance of the dumbbells while the core, hamstrings, and glutes work against gravity to maintain the bridge pose. If the bridge pose is too difficult to maintain for the entire set, one or both partners can drop their hips toward the floor and assume an incline position.

Position of Exercisers

Note that both partners exercise at the same time.

◆ Both exercisers begin seated back-to-back on the floor with dumbbells in each hand.

◆ A stability ball is positioned between the backs of both partners.

◆ Partners slowly roll onto the ball by lifting their hips off the floor while keeping their head and shoulders on the ball.

◆ Partners position feet directly under their knees.

◆ Partners' heads are next to each other.

◆ Bodies should be in a bridge position; head and shoulders are on the ball and hips are lifted into the air.

◆ Hands are positioned over the shoulders.

Movement

◆ Partners begin by drawing their belly buttons in to their spines and squeezing their gluteals to maintain spinal stability.

◆ Partners slowly press dumbbells straight up, extending the arms.

◆ Dumbbells remain positioned over the shoulders during the entire exercise.

◆ Once arms are extended but not locked out, slowly return to the starting position.

Push-Up on Stability Ball

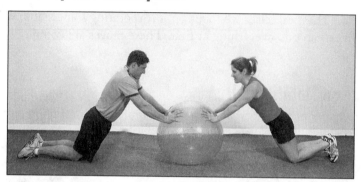

Start/finish.

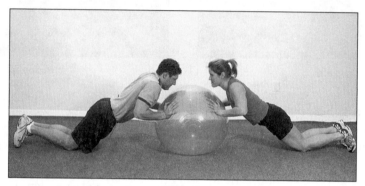

Midpoint.

Push-ups are always a great exercise for strengthening the upper body, especially the chest and triceps. With this exercise, you get the added benefit of abdominal and lower-back strengthening as you use these muscles to stabilize your torso during the exercise. Doing this exercise on the ball creates an extra balance challenge, so if it gets too difficult, put your hands on the ground and keep pushing!

Position of Exercisers

Note that both partners exercise at the same time.

◆ Partners begin by kneeling face-to-face with a stability ball between them.

◆ Partners place their hands on the opposite sides of the ball.

◆ Partners shift their weight forward onto the ball.

◆ Anchoring the feet into the floor, partners extend their hips and knees, moving into a plank position on the ball.

Movement

◆ Simultaneously, partners begin bending their elbows and lowering their chests to the ball.

◆ Slowly, partners extend the arms and return to the starting position.

Chest Press with Tube on Ball with Rotation

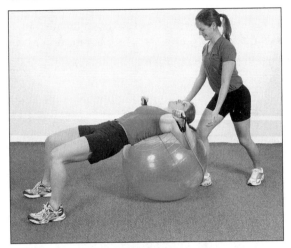

Start/finish.

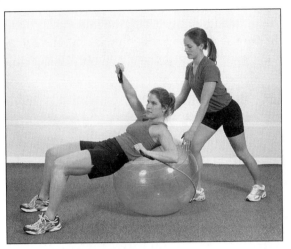

Midpoint.

Now that's a mouthful. A long name usually means that a lot of muscles are working in the exercise. For this particular exercise, the pectoral and shoulder muscles are working to perform the chest press action. In addition, the abdominals are challenged as you move through the torso rotation. If the abdominals begin to fatigue, eliminate the rotation movement and continue with the chest press.

Position of Exerciser

- The exerciser begins seated on the ball holding the handles of an exercise tube in each hand.
- The tube is positioned around the back of the exerciser.
- Slowly roll down into a supine position on the ball.
- Position the ball comfortably between the shoulders and the hips.

Position of Spotter

- The spotter kneels behind the head of the exerciser.
- Step on the center of the tube with one foot to create the anchor for the resistance.

Movement

- Begin by drawing your belly button toward your spine to activate the abdominals.
- Begin by pressing the right hand toward the ceiling, extending the arm.
- Continue the movement by naturally rotating the torso, reaching the arm diagonally across the body.
- While rotating, slightly lift the back off the ball to activate the core muscles.
- Slowly lower back to the starting position.
- Repeat the movement with the other arm.

Back

We're getting creative with the intermediate back workout. Notice how many of these exercises use the core as the stabilizing muscles and the back muscles as the primary movers. Once again, don't be too eager to tackle the whole move at once. Break it down and do what you can.

Lat Pull on Ball

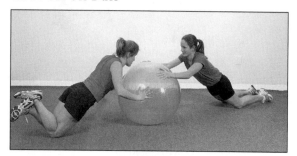

Start/finish.

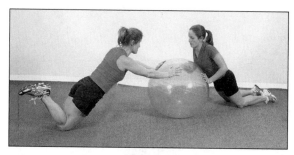

Midpoint.

This exercise not only challenges the latissimus dorsi muscles of the back, but also all of the muscles of the core. We have placed this exercise in the beginning section, but it can be challenging to maintain proper form throughout the entire exercise. Partners must be able to stabilize their core for this exercise. To decrease the intensity, partners can perform the exercise alone on the ball.

Position of Exercisers

Note that both partners exercise at the same time.

◆ Both partners begin by kneeling on the floor with a ball between them.

◆ Both partners hinge forward from the knees, leaning on the ball, keeping arms slightly bent.

Movement

◆ Both partners begin by drawing the belly button in toward the spine to stabilize the core.

◆ To begin the exercise, one partner draws the arms in, bending at the elbows and squeezing the shoulder blades in to the spine.

◆ At the same time, the other partner extends the arms, extending from the shoulders and hips.

◆ To change positions, the partner with the bent arms begins to straighten her arms while the partner with straight arms begins bending at the elbows and retracting the shoulder blades in toward the spine.

Bent Over Row with Tubing and Dumbbells

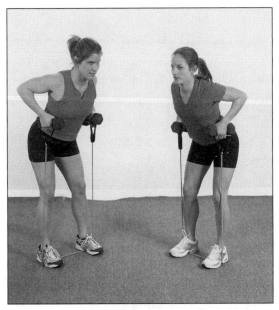

Start/finish.

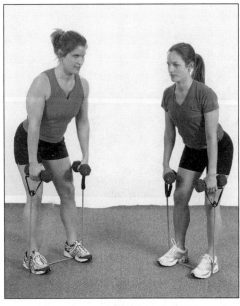

Midpoint.

When an exercise utilizes two different forms of resistance, we call it an integrated exercise. In this exercise, we integrate tubing and dumbbells to create extra resistance for the latissimus dorsi muscles. If at any point during the exercise it becomes too difficult, partners can drop the tubing and continue the exercise with just the dumbbells.

Position of Exerciser

◆ Stand tall with dumbbells in each hand and the handle ends of an exercise tube in each hand.

◆ Step on the middle of the tube with both feet.

◆ Hinge at the hips, positioning your body as pictured.

◆ Be sure to keep the spine long and the back flat.

Movement

◆ Begin by drawing your belly button in toward your spine to stabilize the torso.

◆ With both arm extended straight down to the floor, keep elbows in toward your sides and draw arms up to the ceiling.

◆ Squeeze shoulder blades into the spine.

◆ Slowly lower to the starting position.

Back Extension on Stability Ball with Medicine Ball

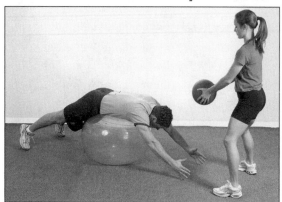

Start/finish.

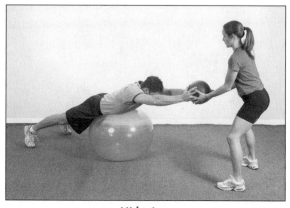

Midpoint.

This back extension exercise is similar to the one we did in the beginner workout, except we've added the balance and resistance dimensions with the stability ball and medicine ball. In this exercise, the spotting partner is there to give a target to the exerciser as he lifts the medicine ball. Partners need to communicate to determine how high the exerciser can lift. To lessen the resistance, partners can do this exercise without the medicine ball.

Position of Exerciser

◆ The exerciser begins by lying prone on a stability ball with his feet extended behind him and belly button centered over the ball.

◆ Hold a medicine ball in both hands, with arms extended in front of you.

◆ To stabilize yourself, position your feet about 3 feet apart.

Position of Spotter

◆ Stand at the head of the exerciser, approximately 3 feet from the exerciser's head.

◆ Extend your arms, giving the spotter a target to lift the medicine ball to.

Movement

◆ Contract the lower back and slowly lift the chest and arms.

◆ Raise the medicine ball up to the spotter's target.

◆ Touch the medicine ball to your partner's hands and then slowly lower back to the starting position.

Arms

Like many of the other exercises in this section, we have added challenges to some regular arm-strengthening exercises to make them more difficult. Always remember that you can revert to the simplified exercise whenever you need to.

Tube Curls on Stability Balls

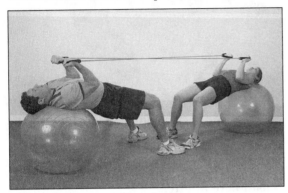

Start/finish.

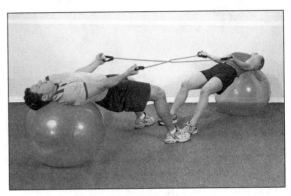

Midpoint.

This exercise is simply a traditional bicep curl, except that we've positioned you lying on a stability ball. This new position will challenge the legs and core while slightly changing the angle of the arm to produce a great bicep workout. The distance between the partners will determine the resistance on the tubes. For starters, begin positioned close to your partner. As you improve, you can put more space between you to make the exercise more challenging.

Position of Exercisers

Note that both partners exercise at the same time.

◆ Twist two tubes together, with both partners holding on to the handles of a single tube.

◆ Both partners begin seated on separate stability balls holding on to their tubes.

◆ Partners slowly recline so that their backs are on the ball.

◆ If this position is too strenuous on either partner's neck, they can come closer together and place their heads on the ball.

◆ Partners' arms should be extended straight out toward their knees.

Movement

◆ While stabilizing their spines, partners slowly flex their elbows, drawing their hands in to their shoulders.

◆ The resistance on the tube will increase as you pull.

◆ Once elbows are completely flexed, slowly extend the arms and return to the starting position.

Kneeling Triceps Extension

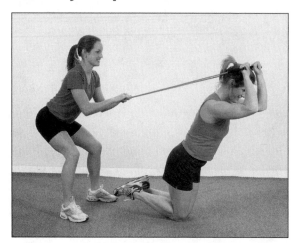

Start/finish.

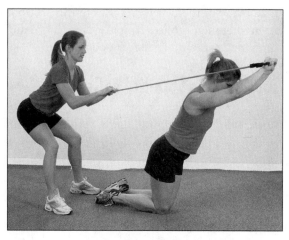

Midpoint.

This triceps exercise can be challenging for both the spotter and the exerciser. As you can see from the picture, the kneeling partner works the triceps, while the spotting partner works the legs and glutes in the squatting position. This is a double-trouble exercise. Once again, the resistance on the tube is determined by the distance between the partners. Start close and add distance as you improve.

Position of Exerciser

- Begin by grasping the handles of a tube, keeping the loop of the tube behind you for the spotter to hold.

- Kneel on the floor with your hands above your head and your elbows pointed to the wall in front of you.

- Keep the spine straight and hinge slightly forward from the knees so your body is angled slightly toward the wall in front of you.

Position of Spotter

- Position yourself behind the exerciser and grasp the loop of the tube with both hands.

- With your arms extended in front of you, slowly lower your hips down into a squatting position.

Movement

- The exerciser extends both arms, pressing the hands toward the wall in front of her.

- Keep the torso stabilized as you extend.

- Once arms are completely extended, slowly flex the elbows and return to the starting position.

Stability Ball Dips

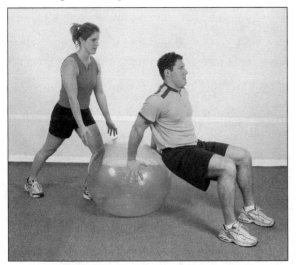

Start/finish.

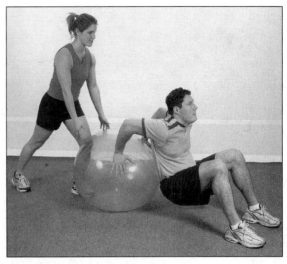

Midpoint.

In the beginner workout, we started you and your partner out with dips on a bench or a chair. In this intermediate workout, we make it more challenging by having you perform the same exercise on an unsteady stability ball. Not only are your arms working hard, but so are your abdominals to keep you from sliding around.

Position of Exerciser

Note that both partners exercise at the same time.

◆ Begin by sitting tall on the ball.
◆ Place hands on the ball directly behind your hips.
◆ Legs are extended out away from the ball but knees remain slightly bent.

Movement

◆ Begin by pressing your hands into the ball and lifting your hips up off the ball.
◆ Scoot hips slightly forward so they are no longer directly on top of the ball.
◆ Bending at the elbows, slowly lower your hips toward the floor.
◆ When elbows are bent to 90 degrees, slowly extend arms, returning to the starting position.

Bicep Curl with Tube and Weights

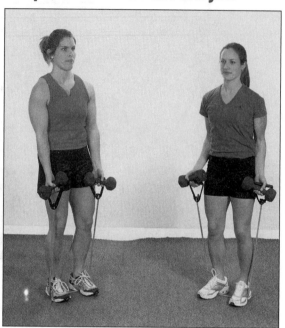

Start/finish.

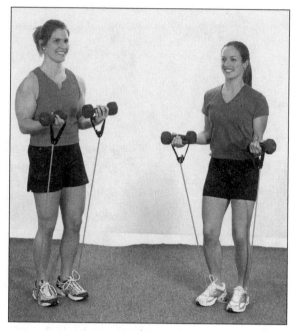

Midpoint.

This is another integrated exercise designed to provide an extra challenge for the bicep muscles of the upper arm. If the exercise becomes too difficult, drop the tube handles and continue the exercise with just the dumbbells in hand. If you want to increase the resistance, spread your feet apart, creating less "gap" for the tube.

Position of Exercisers

◆ Both partners begin with exercise tube handles and dumbbells in each hand.

◆ Both partners stand on the middle of their own exercise tube.

◆ Standing tall with arms extended at their sides, both partners draw their belly buttons in towards their spines for spinal support.

◆ Elbows are anchored to the hips and shoulders are pulling away from the ears.

Movement

◆ Slowly flex the elbows, curling the hands up toward the shoulders.

◆ Pull hands all the way in toward the shoulders.

◆ Slowly extend the arms and return to the starting position.

Shoulders

We hope your arms aren't too tired, because you still have several shoulder exercises to get through before your workout is complete. Each of these exercises incorporates the shoulder muscles along with some other muscle group in the body. All of this multidimensional training will have you fit in no time!

Lateral Raise Side-Lying on Stability Ball

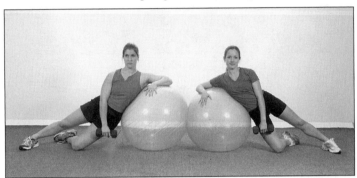

Start/finish.

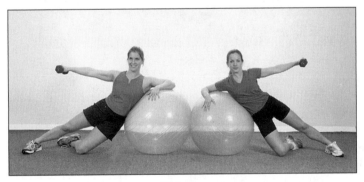

Midpoint.

This exercise looks and feels easy at first, but keep going. While your shoulder grows tired from the lateral raises, your gluteals will be begging for mercy as they are engaged the entire time to stabilize you on the ball. As an added bonus, your abdominals and lower back are working hard to keep you in the proper position.

Position of Exercisers

Note that both partners exercise at the same time.

◆ Both partners begin by side-lying on a stability ball with a dumbbell in the top hand.

◆ The top arm is extended down to the floor in front of the body.

◆ The bottom knee is on the floor and the top leg is extended straight out.

Movement

◆ Draw your belly button in toward your spine to stabilize the core.

◆ Slowly raise the top hand toward the ceiling, keeping arm extended.

◆ When arm reaches shoulder height, slowly lower back down to the starting position.

Stork Stance

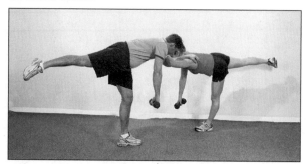

Start/finish.

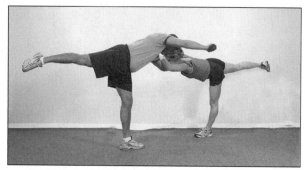

Midpoint.

The stork stance refers to the position of the body during this exercise. In this position, you engage the leg muscles to keep you balanced, your core to keep you stabilized, and of course your shoulders to perform the raise. You can make this movement more difficult by separating from your partner and performing the exercise on your own. Or to simplify things, use the wall for a more stable support.

Position of Exerciser

Note that both partners exercise at the same time.

- Both partners begin by facing each other with their inside shoulders lined up.
- Partners hold one dumbbell in their outside hand.
- Partners place their inside hands on each other's inside shoulder with arms completely extended.

- Both partners hinge at their hips and slowly lower their chests to the floor while they lift their outside legs to the ceiling.
- The outside leg rises to a level so that it is parallel to the floor.
- The outside arm, with dumbbell in hand, is extended toward the floor.

Movement

- Holding on to your partner's arm for support, draw your belly button in to your spine to stabilize the core.
- Slowly raise your arm forward.
- Keep eyes focused on the floor to maintain spinal alignment and balance.
- When arm is parallel to the floor, slowly lower arm back to the starting position.

Shoulder Press with Tubes on Stability Ball

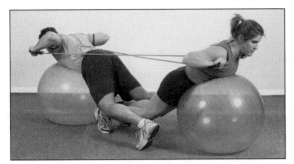

Start/finish.

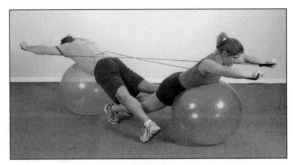

Midpoint.

In the beginning workout, we did a shoulder press seated on stability balls. In this intermediate workout, we've made the same exercise more challenging by changing the body position and method of resistance. This shoulder press exercise will not only work the shoulder muscles, but also the core as you stabilize your torso during the exercise. If it is too challenging for partners to perform the exercise at the same time, one partner can press while the other holds.

Position of Exercisers

Note that both partners exercise at the same time.

◆ Twist two tubes together with each partner holding the handles of a single tube.

◆ Both partners position themselves prone on stability balls facing away from each other with their feet touching.

◆ Begin with hands in front of shoulders, elbows flexed.

Movement

◆ Partners begin by extending the arms straight out in front of their shoulders, keeping arms parallel to the ground.

◆ Once the arms are fully extended, but not locked out, slowly flex the elbows and return to the starting position.

The Least You Need to Know

◆ The intermediate workout has many levels to accommodate a partner who is progressing more slowly than the other partner.

◆ Change the order of the exercises often. This will keep your muscles guessing.

◆ If the compound exercises are too difficult, consider doing only one of the movements when you first begin.

◆ You can go back to exercises from Chapter 13 when your muscles need a break.

In This Chapter

◆ How to take easy moves and make them more challenging through balance and stabilization

◆ Advanced exercises for a total body workout

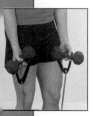
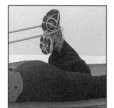
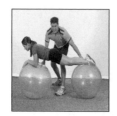
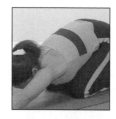
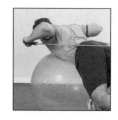
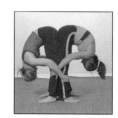

Chapter 15

Work It Out: Advanced

Congratulations on achieving yet another level of fitness. By progressing to the advanced workout, you have proved your dedication to your fitness adventure. You and your partner must be feeling and looking great by now and the extra challenge of this advanced workout will help to keep your motivation and momentum up.

In this chapter, we'll be taking you through another total body strength-training workout. These advanced exercises have more balance and stability challenges than any of our other workout programs, so get ready to work. For a slow transition from the intermediate workouts, pay attention to the tips we give you for progression.

Now let's do it!

The Basics

What tips can we give folks of your awesome fitness ability? After all, if you made it to this chapter, you must know just about everything by now! So let's use this section of the chapter to remind you of a few things you may have forgotten as you've grown from beginner to advanced.

- **Don't Leave Your Partner Behind.** Once you get to the advanced workouts, it's tempting to progress without your partner, especially if one of you is more ready than the other. Don't forget that we have designed many of our exercises so that one partner can do a higher intensity version and one partner can do a lower one. You don't need to progress at the same time. Both of you just need to keep improving.

- **Too Many Moving Parts Can Spell Trouble.** Many of these exercises involve some kind of balance or stability challenge in addition to the traditional movement of the exercises. Moving multiple joints at the same time can be tricky, so proceed with caution. It's best to get the main movement down first, and then progress to the secondary movements as you improve.

- **Bat Out of Order.** Each muscle group contains three to four different exercises. However you don't have to do those exercises in the order that we've laid them out in the book. Instead change the order around with each workout to keep it interesting for your muscles. If you always do the same exercise last, chances are you will always be too tired to do it properly. So to get the most from each workout, change it up often.

- **Sore No More.** You wish. We know we don't need to remind you of this, but prepare yourself for more muscle soreness as you tackle this new workout. The good news is that you will probably recover from your soreness quicker because you are in such great shape!

Tools of the Trade

Great news! No more equipment to buy. You have everything you're going to need for this advanced workout already (if you purchased everything we recommended in earlier chapters). Here's a complete list of what you should have by now:

- Exercise Mat
- Stability Balls (two)
- Dumbbells (varying weights)
- Exercise Tubes (two)
- Medicine Ball

If you have all of these, you're ready to go.

The Workout

Now that you are an advanced strength-training exerciser, you can start to challenge the muscles with not only more resistance and heavier weights, but also balance, stabilization, and agility. Remember, fitness is not just about strength, but about how your body can react and adapt to the challenges that are placed on it. This advanced workout incorporates all of those dimensions in a fun and effective program that you and your partner will both enjoy.

Let's check it out.

Core

Once again, your core muscles are the focal point of this workout. Without strength in your abdominals and lower back, you won't be able to perform any of the other exercises in this chapter properly. These core exercises are challenging and should be attempted with caution for those partners who have lower back issues or injuries.

Partner Stability Ball Toss from Hands to Feet

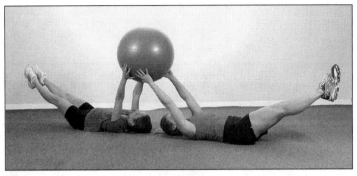

Start/finish.

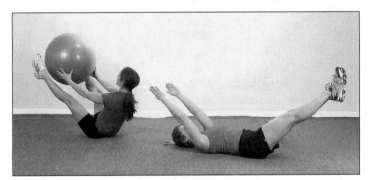

Midpoint.

Looks like fun, doesn't it? In this exercise, the partners are engaging the upper and lower portions of the abdominals as they pass the ball from their hands to their feet. If the stability ball is too heavy or awkward for either partner, a medicine ball can be substituted.

Position of Exercisers

Note that both partners exercise at the same time.

- ◆ Both partners begin by lying supine on the floor, head to head with their legs extended.
- ◆ Place your arms over your head. There should be enough distance between you so that when your arms are extended, your hands touch your partner's hands.
- ◆ One partner will begin holding the ball between her feet.

Movement

- ◆ The partner with the ball begins with her feet on the ground, the ball between her feet.
- ◆ As she lifts the ball up to the ceiling, she lifts her upper body, reaching her hands toward the ball.
- ◆ In this position, she passes the ball from her feet to her hands.
- ◆ As she begins to lower her body down to the floor, she extends the ball over her head and passes it to her partner's hands.
- ◆ The other partner follows the same motion in the opposite order, passing the ball from her hands to her feet.
- ◆ Partners continue passing the ball back and forth to each other.

Prone Plank on Two Stability Balls

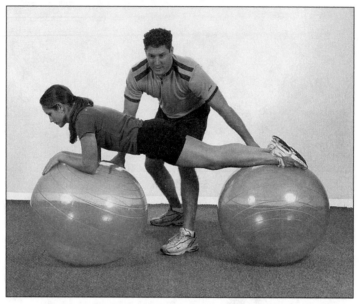

This exercise is extremely challenging for the core muscles, but is not recommended for individuals with lower back injuries.

This is another isometric exercise designed to strengthen all of the muscles in the core. With elbows and feet on the ball, the balance challenge is increased, requiring the exercising partner to engage all of the core muscles. If a third ball is available, partners can do this exercise at the same time by putting their elbows on the same ball and their feet on separate balls. This exercise is not recommended for individuals with lower back injuries.

Position of Exerciser

◆ The exercising partner begins by kneeling on the floor with his elbow on a stability ball.

◆ The spotter assists the exerciser in lifting the feet on to the stability ball.

◆ In this position, the exerciser will have his elbows on one ball and his feet on another.

Position of Spotter

◆ The spotter positions himself near the midsection of the exerciser.

◆ Position your hands so that you are able to stabilize the exerciser's hips if she starts to wobble or move.

Movement

◆ The exerciser holds this position for as long as she can without falling off either ball.

Reverse Curl on Stability Ball

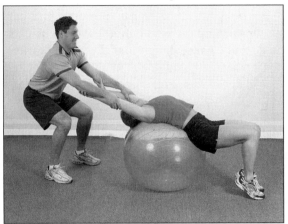

Start/finish.

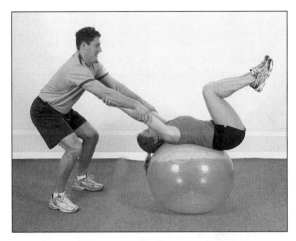

Midpoint.

This reverse curl is a challenging exercise for the hard-to-reach lower portion of the abdominals. Partners take turns performing this exercise, but as you can see from the photo, both partners exercise at the same time. The partner on the ball strengthens the abdominals while the spotter engages the legs and glutes in the squat position. Another double-trouble exercise!

Position of the Exerciser

◆ The exerciser begins by lying on a stability ball with her arms extended over her head and feet on the ground.

◆ Grasping the outstretched hands of the spotter, lift your feet several inches off the ground.

Position of the Spotter

◆ Extend your arms out, grasping the wrists of your partner.

◆ Slowly lower yourself into a squat position.

Movement

◆ The exerciser slowly curls her knees into her chest, curling the lower back off the ball.

◆ Slowly return to the starting position, with your feet several inches off the floor.

◆ Try not to let your feet touch the floor between repetitions.

Legs

Welcome to a powerful leg workout. With these exercises, you can expect to gain not only strength but also power from those sculpted sticks holding up your increasingly well-defined body! The extra challenge with this workout comes from added resistance and balance dimensions. Enjoy the variety and try to add more resistance when you can.

Step-Ups

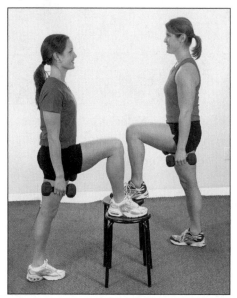

Start/finish.

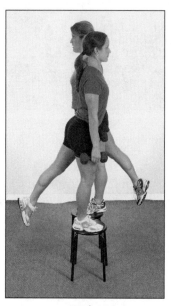

Midpoint.

Step-ups are a great exercise for strengthening all of the muscles in the lower extremity. Primarily, your quadriceps are working as you step up on the bench. As you step back down, the adductors and calves activate to control your movement back to the floor. You can increase the difficulty of this exercise by holding dumbbells in each hand while stepping up.

Position of Exercisers

Note that both partners exercise at the same time.

◆ Begin by choosing a bench or step height that is suitable for both partners. When stepping onto the bench, the knee should not flex more than 90 degrees.

◆ Both partners stand facing the bench or steps with arms at their sides.

Movement

◆ Both partners step up on to the bench, keeping foot and knee pointed forward.

◆ Be sure to place the entire foot on the bench. Do not allow heel to hang off the back of the bench.

◆ Push through the heel as you continue stepping up on the bench, bring the back leg up off the floor.

◆ Continue lifting back leg up, flexing at the hip and knee.

◆ Balance on the standing leg.

◆ Slowly lower the back leg down to the floor and return to the starting position.

◆ Repeat the exercise with the other leg stepping first.

Ball Squat Back-to-Back

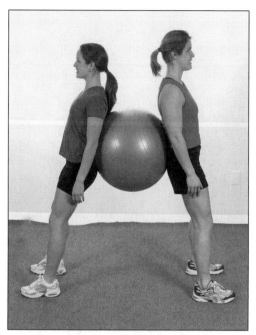

Start/finish.

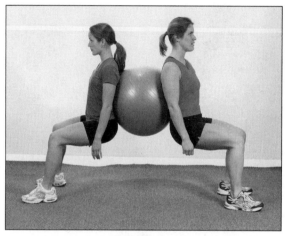

Midpoint.

Squats are an excellent exercise to strengthen the muscles of the quadriceps and gluteals. In this squat exercise, there is the added element of the balance challenge as the partners try to maintain their balance while being supported by a moving object. To complete the exercise effectively, it is helpful if both partners are of similar height and fitness ability. If the balance challenge is too difficult, partners can do this exercise individually by doing it against a wall.

Position of Exercisers

Note that both partners exercise at the same time.

◆ Both partners stand back-to-back.

◆ The stability ball is positioned between the two partners, resting just above their lower backs.

◆ Feet are positioned eight inches out in front of the hips.

◆ Knees and toes are pointed forward and the back is straight.

◆ Partners lean into the ball slightly, using the resistance of their partner for support.

Movement

◆ Partners begin by drawing their belly buttons in toward their spines.

◆ Simultaneously both partners lower their hips toward the floor, into a squat position.

◆ Partners should continue lowering until their knees are bent 90 degrees.

◆ Knees should not extend over the toes.

◆ Weight is pressing through the heels, and not into the toes.

◆ Slowly return to the starting position, keeping weight back on the ball the entire time.

To increase the challenge, partners can hold dumbbells in each hand.

Lunge Forward with Transverse Torque with Tube

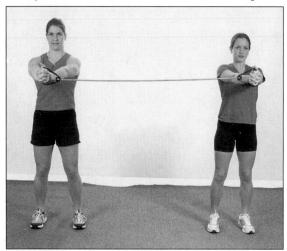

Start/finish.

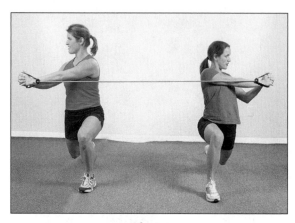

Midpoint.

This exercise is a mouthful to say, and it is complex for the body as well. In this movement, the exerciser works both the muscles of the legs and the core. The resistance is determined by the tension of the tube and the distance between the two partners.

Position of Exerciser

◆ The exerciser stands straight with feet together, facing forward.

◆ The exerciser holds one handle of an exercise tube in both hands.

◆ Arms are extended directly out in front of the exerciser, parallel to the floor.

Position of Spotter

◆ The spotter stands off to the side of the exerciser.

◆ The spotter holds the other handle of the exercise tube with both hands.

◆ Arms are extended directly out in front of the spotter, parallel to the floor.

Movement

◆ The exerciser lunges forward with the outside leg, stepping far enough out so that as you lower your back knee to the floor, the front knee stays over your front ankle.

◆ At the same time, resist against the tension of the tube and turn the shoulders toward the outside of the body.

◆ Be sure to maintain back alignment by keeping your belly button drawn in to your spine and your back straight.

◆ Slowly step feet back together, returning to the starting position.

◆ After completing one set on this side, have your spotter move to the other side and perform the exercise with the other leg lunging forward.

Single-Leg Partner Lunges

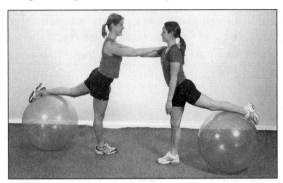

Start/finish.

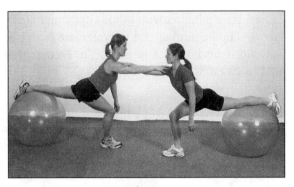

Midpoint.

This single-leg lunge challenges both partners to maintain their balance and stability while strengthening the muscles of the legs and glutes. In these pictures, we illustrate the partners holding on to each other for support. However, as you get stronger and become more stable, you may want to try the exercise without holding on to your partner.

Position of Exercisers

◆ Partners begin by standing facing each other with their inside arms extended, grasping each other's shoulders for support.

◆ Their inside legs are planted on the ground and their outside legs are positioned on top of a stability ball.

◆ Partners should be balancing on their front leg with only minimal weight on the back leg.

Movement

◆ Both partners slowly bend the front knee as they slide their back leg out behind them.

◆ As you lower, focus on keeping the front knee over your ankle, bending that knee only 90 degrees.

◆ Reach the back leg out as far as you can.

◆ Keep the back straight as you lower, trying not to hinge forward as you lower to the ground.

◆ Slowly return to the starting position.

Chest

The advanced chest workout is all about stability and control throughout the chest and shoulder areas. The beginning and intermediate exercises have prepared you for the extra challenges in this advanced workout. It's important to execute these exercises slowly so you can get the maximum benefit from each movement.

Stability Ball Chest Fly

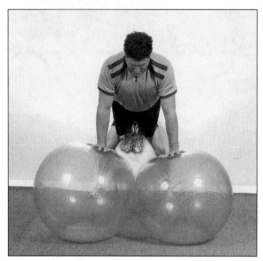

Start/finish.

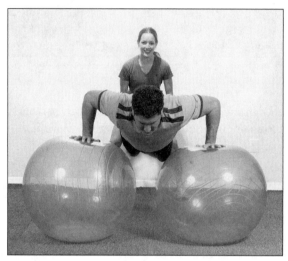

Midpoint.

This super exercise for the chest requires abdominal and lower back strength. You can begin doing this exercise as we describe it here. As you improve, you can put your hands on the ball for an extra balance challenge. If it's too difficult to do with your legs up, start with them on the floor.

Position of the Spotter

◆ Begin by kneeling on the floor with two stability balls in front of you.

◆ Place your forearms on each stability ball, keeping your elbows close to your sides.

◆ Extend your legs behind you.

Position of Exerciser

◆ Stand behind your partner, at his feet.

◆ Reach down and pick up your partner's feet, lifting them until his legs are parallel to the ground.

Movement

◆ The exerciser begins pushing the arms out to the sides, keeping the elbows bent.

◆ As the balls roll out the sides, the exerciser lowers his chest down to the floor.

◆ When your body is completely parallel to the floor, slowly return to the starting position by drawing the elbows in to your sides and your forearms back under you.

Push-Up with Medicine Ball Roll

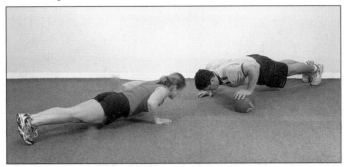

Start/finish.

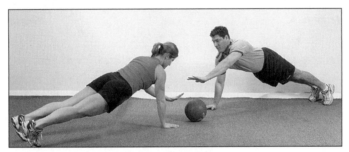

Midpoint.

Not just your average push-up! Push-ups on a medicine ball will stretch the shoulder muscles as you strengthen the chest. Rolling the ball back and forth between partners is a great way to challenge your coordination and agility. You can do this exercise on your knees or on your feet depending on your ability.

Position of Exercisers

◆ Both partners begin by facing each other in a push-up position.

◆ Partners can be positioned on their knees or on their feet and both partners don't have to be in the same position to perform the exercise.

◆ One partner begins with a medicine ball under one hand.

Movement

◆ Both partners lower their chests to the floor, bending at the elbows.

◆ On the way back up, the partner with the ball rolls it diagonally across to her partner's opposite hand.

◆ Both partners perform a push-up again.

◆ Partners pass the ball back and forth between push-ups.

◆ Do the same thing with the ball in the other hand.

Decline Dumbbell Chest Press Plank on Stability Ball

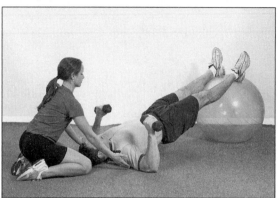

Start/finish.

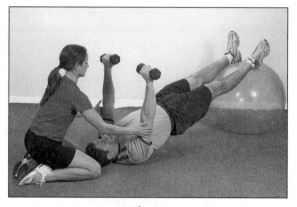

Midpoint.

Decline chest presses help to strengthen the muscles in the lower part of the pectoral region. Performing this exercise plank on a ball also engages the abs and lower back. Even the legs are working to stabilize you. This is a total body exercise!

Position of Exerciser

◆ The exerciser begins by lying supine on the floor with his feet on a stability ball.

◆ With dumbbells in each hand, position your hands over your shoulders with the back of your arm and elbow on the ground.

◆ Slowly lift your hips off the ground into a plank position.

Position of Spotter

◆ Assist your partner by stabilizing the ball as he moves into the starting position.

◆ Once he is stabilized, stand behind your partner's head and spot him from the elbows as he lifts the weight.

Movement

◆ From the plank position with hips lifted, slowly extend the arms, pressing the dumbbells toward the ceiling.

◆ When arms are fully extended but not locked out, return to the starting position.

Back

Before you can successfully achieve the sculpted look of a Greek god, you've got to make it through this advanced back workout. These exercises will help to continue to define the muscles we've been working on in the other workouts. Take your time to execute these exercises slowly and with proper form. While the resistance is not that great, the challenge in these exercises comes from your ability to perform them properly. Encourage your partner to focus on feeling the back muscles working in each exercise.

Stork Stance Lat Pull with Tube

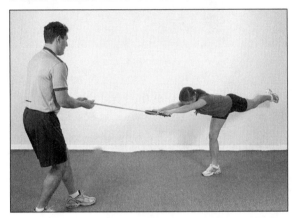

Start/finish.

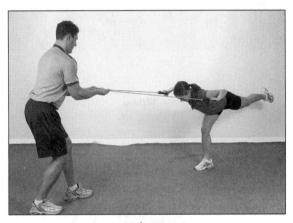

Midpoint.

Most exercisers are familiar with the lat pull exercise commonly performed on machines. This exercise is a variation, only it is executed in a stork stance, semiprone, with a tube. The resistance level will depend on the tension of the tube and the distance between the tube partners.

Position of Exerciser

◆ Grasp the handles of the tube in each hand.

◆ With one leg planted firmly on the ground, slowly extend the back leg behind you and raise it off the ground.

◆ As you raise your leg, lower your chest and torso toward the floor. Stop when your head and foot are in a straight line, parallel to the floor.

◆ Extend your arms straight out in front of you.

Position of Spotter

◆ Grasp the middle loop of the tube with both hands.

◆ Stand far enough away from your partner to create light resistance on the tube.

Movement

◆ Begin with arms extended and palms facing the floor.

◆ The exerciser slowly pulls the handles of the tube toward her shoulders, squeezing the shoulders down into the spine as she pulls.

◆ After the range of motion is complete, slowly extend the arms, returning to the starting position.

Bent Over Reverse Fly on Ball

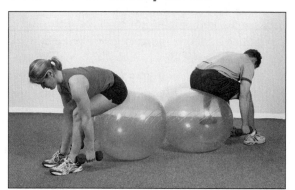

Start/finish.

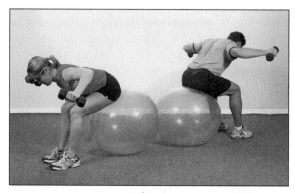

Midpoint.

This exercise is designed to strengthen the back portion of the shoulder and upper back muscles. If a ball is not available, partners can perform the exercise seated in a chair or on a bench. The focus of the exercise should be on squeezing the shoulder blades together as you lift. To decrease the resistance, partners should keep their elbows bent as they lift.

Position of Exercisers

Note that both partners exercise at the same time.

◆ Both partners begin seated on the ball with dumbbells in each hand.

◆ Feet are flat on the floor and knees and toes are pointed forward.

◆ Hinge forward at the hips, lowering your chest down toward your knees.

◆ Maintain spinal alignment by keeping the back flat and the neck long and extended.

◆ Arms begin extended straight to the floor, placed slightly behind the ankles.

Movement

◆ Keeping the chest close to the knees, slowly raise arms to the ceiling, keeping the arms straight.

◆ Continue lifting arms to the ceiling while squeezing your shoulder blades together in the back.

◆ Once arms are parallel to the floor, lower to the starting position.

Back Extension Ball Toss

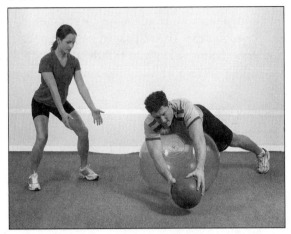

Start/finish.

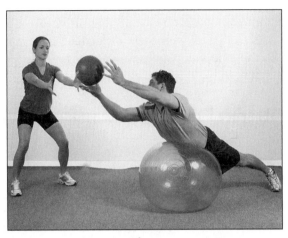

Midpoint.

We've stepped up the traditional back extension one more notch. In this exercise, the spotting partner will be tossing a medicine ball to the exercising partner. As the exerciser goes through the range of motion, she will be tossing the ball back to the spotter. This motion engages all of the muscles of the back and arms, as well as the core. To get the hang of the motion, try it a few times without the ball.

Position of Exerciser

◆ Begin by lying prone on a ball with your legs extended behind you and your arms in front of the ball.

◆ To maintain stability, position your feet about 3 feet apart.

◆ Begin with your chest lifted slightly off the ball.

Position of Spotter

◆ Stand off to one side of your partner holding a medicine ball in your hands.

◆ Position yourself about 4 feet away from your partner.

Movement

◆ The exerciser begins by turning her head and arms to the spotter.

◆ The spotter gently tosses the ball into the exerciser's hands.

◆ The exerciser completes the range of motion by lowering her chest down to the ball and swinging her arms in a downward motion away from the spotter.

◆ On the way back up, the exerciser looks toward the spotter and tosses the ball back to her.

◆ Repeat this exercise with the spotter on the other side.

Arms

Is it time to transform your guns into heavy artillery? This arm workout combines some basic exercises from earlier chapters with a few added challenges. Try to increase the resistance on the exercises by using heavier dumbbells or stronger tubes. When using the ball, go slow and feel the muscles working.

Stability Ball Triceps Extension with Tube

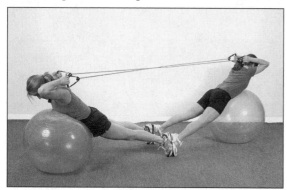

Start/finish.

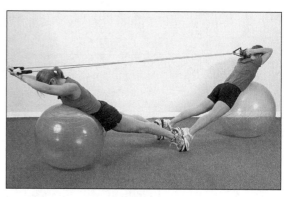

Midpoint.

This exercise is similar to one we illustrated in the beginner strength workout. In the previous chapter, the triceps extension with tube was executed from a standing position. With this exercise, you are prone on a stability ball. Your lower back muscles will be working to stabilize your upper body for the triceps extension. This is a great added challenge! If the resistance of the tube is too tight, partners can perform the exercise one at a time. While one partner extends the arms, the other partner's arms can remain flexed to lessen the tension.

Position of Exercisers

Note that both partners exercise at the same time.

◆ Twist two tubes together, with each partner grasping the handles of a single tube.

◆ Partners begin by lying prone over a stability ball with their feet touching and their heads facing away from each other.

◆ Partners position their arms as indicated in the picture with elbows pointing forward and hands behind their heads.

Movement

◆ Partners simultaneously extend arms, pressing hands forward.

◆ Once arms are completely extended, slowly flex the elbows and return to the starting position.

Dips on Two Stability Balls

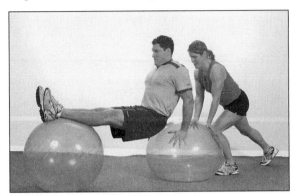

Start/finish.

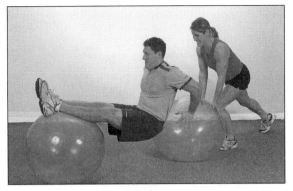

Midpoint.

Talk about a balance challenge! This exercise requires the exercisers to have a strong core, good arm strength, and adequate balance. If it's too challenging at first, start with just your hands on the ball. Progress to the feet on the ball when your arms and core can support and stabilize you. In this exercise, the spotter is positioned to catch you if you fall!

Position of Exerciser

◆ It's easiest to begin seated on one stability ball with your hands positioned behind your hips.

◆ Slowly lift both feet onto the other ball, one foot at a time.

◆ Stay seated on the first ball until your partner is in position to spot you.

Position of Spotter

◆ Stand directly behind the exerciser with your hands close to the ball that her hands are on.

◆ If the exerciser looks wobbly, position your hands on the ball to steady her.

Movement

◆ Lift your hips off the ball and slide them slightly forward.

◆ Bending only at the elbows, lower your hips down toward the floor, or until your elbows are bent 90 degrees.

◆ Pushing your hands into the ball, slowly extend the arms back to the starting position.

Stork Stance Arm Curl

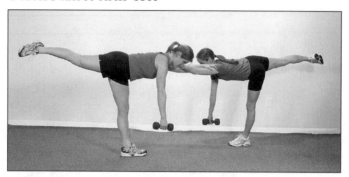

Start/finish.

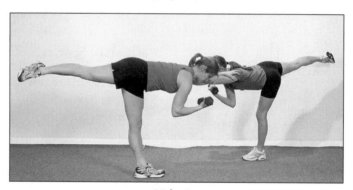

Midpoint.

The stork stance is back again! By performing the bicep curl in a stork stance you eliminate the ability to cheat by using your back to help you lift the weight. In this position, you isolate the arm so that only the bicep can do the work. As with all stork stance exercises, you can try it without holding on to your partner for support as you improve your balance.

Position of the Exerciser

Note that both partners exercise at the same time.

- Both partners begin by facing each other with their inside shoulders lined up.
- Partners hold one dumbbell in their outside hand.
- Partners place their inside hands on each other's inside shoulder with arms completely extended.

- Both partners hinge at their hips and slowly lower their chests to the floor while they lift their outside legs to the ceiling.
- The outside leg rises to a level so that it is parallel to the floor.
- The outside arm, with dumbbell in hand, is extended toward the floor.

Movement

- Holding on to your partner's arm for support, draw your belly button in to your spine to stabilize the core.
- Slowly flex your elbow, curling your hand up toward your shoulder.
- Keep eyes focused on the floor to maintain spinal alignment and balance.
- When arm is completely flexed, slowly extend the arm and return to the starting position.

Manual Resistance Bicep Curls with Dumbbells

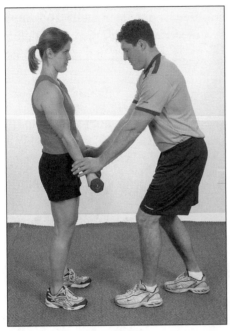

Start/finish.

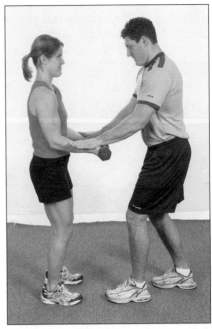

Midpoint.

And you thought manual resistance exercises were only for beginners! No way! This manual resistance exercise is tough and you may just have to try it to believe us. Use lighter hand weights with this at first. Your partner will be adding the extra resistance so you don't have to go real heavy from the start.

Position of Exerciser

◆ The exerciser begins by standing with feet hip-width apart and back straight.

◆ Keep arms extended down to your sides with dumbbells in each hand.

◆ Keep your shoulders retracted and not hunched.

Position of Spotter

◆ Position yourself facing your partner about 1 foot apart.

◆ Place your hands on your partner's forearms, midway between the wrist and elbow.

◆ As the exerciser lifts, you will be applying downward pressure.

Movement

◆ As the spotter applies downward pressure, the exerciser flexes at the elbow, curling the weights up to the shoulders.

◆ Once the elbow is completely flexed, the spotter will continue pushing down on the exerciser's arms.

◆ As the exerciser extends his arms back to the starting position, he will resist against the force of the spotter.

Shoulders

Your advanced workout would not be complete without some creative shoulder exercises. The shoulders are key to completing your total body workout and these exercises are designed to compliment the other upper body exercises in this program. As always, focus on form first, and add the resistance as you improve.

Rear Deltoid Row on Ball

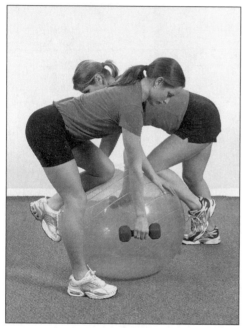

Start/finish.

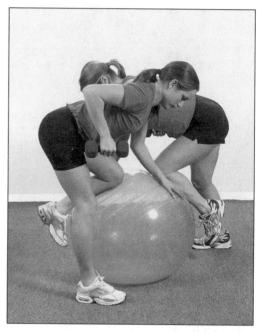

Midpoint.

Don't be fooled. This exercise only looks easy. In this exercise, the standing leg is working to stabilize the weight of the upper body while the abdominals and lower back secure the torso.

Position of Exercisers

Note that both partners exercise at the same time.

- Both partners begin by facing each other with a ball between them.
- Partners hold one dumbbell in their outside hand.
- Partners place their inside hands and their inside knee on the ball, bending forward slightly to support the weight of their body.

- The outside arm, with dumbbell in hand, is extended toward the floor.

Movement

- Pressing down into the ball for support, draw your belly button in to your spine to stabilize the core.
- Slowly pull your arm back, flexing at the elbow.
- Keep eyes focused on the floor to maintain spinal alignment and balance.
- Lower arm back to the starting position.

Kneeling Stability Ball Manual Resistance Lateral Raise

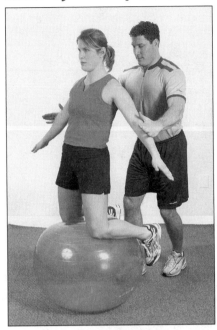

Start/finish.

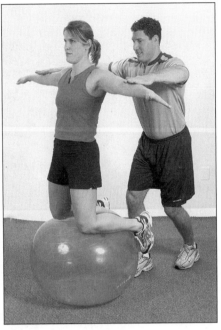

Midpoint.

That's a mouthful! This exercise is hard to say and equally as difficult to perform. This shoulder exercise is actually a total body challenge. While the core works to stabilize you, the arms are challenged by your partner's manual resistance. The balance is probably the hardest part of this exercise, so use your partner for support as you begin this exercise.

Position of Exerciser

◆ Begin by standing behind the ball.
◆ Place your hands on the ball and then place one knee on the ball at a time.
◆ Get your balance. If you need to, use your partner to stabilize you.
◆ Once you are balanced, lengthen your spine to a full kneeling position and extend your arms out to the side.

Position of Spotter

◆ Stand directly behind your partner and help to stabilize him if he needs it.
◆ Place your hands on the exerciser's forearms, just below his elbow.
◆ Begin to apply downward pressure on your partner's arms.

Movement

◆ As the spotter pushes the exerciser's arms down, the exerciser resists.
◆ Keeping the arms straight, the exerciser continues to lift the arms as the spotter pushes them down.
◆ When the exerciser's arms are down at his sides, the exerciser lifts them back, pressing against the resistance of the spotter.

Stork Stance Scapulation

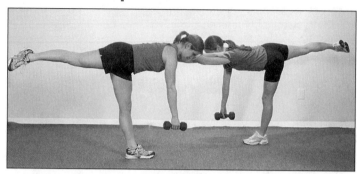

Start/finish.

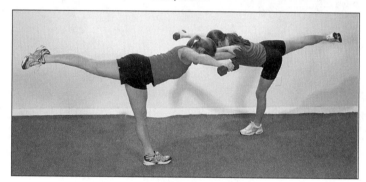

Midpoint.

Scapulation refers to the angle the arm is lifted in this exercise. Scapulation is lifting diagonally away from the body. Just imagine a front raise and a lateral raise. With scapulation, you are lifting in between those two ranges of motion. In this exercise, lift diagonally away from your body, keeping your arm straight. As your balance improves, try to do this without holding on to your partner.

Position of Exerciser

Note that both partners exercise at the same time.

- Both partners begin by facing each other with their inside shoulders lined up.
- Partners hold one dumbbell in their outside hand.
- Partners place their inside hands on each other's inside shoulder, arms completely extended.

- Both partners hinge at their hips and slowly lower chests to the floor while they lift their outside legs to the ceiling.
- The outside leg rises to a level so that it is parallel to the floor.
- The outside arm, with dumbbell in hand, is extended toward the floor.

Movement

- Holding on to your partner's arm for support, draw your belly button in to your spine to stabilize the core.
- Slowly extend your arm diagonally out away from your body, lifting it toward the ceiling.
- Keep eyes focused on the floor to maintain spinal alignment and balance.
- When your arm is parallel to the floor, slowly lower it back down to the starting position.

The Least You Need to Know

- Advanced strength training does not necessarily mean lifting heavier weights.
- Changing the order of your exercise routine will keep your muscles engaged and will fight off boredom.
- With a few small changes, both partners can enjoy this workout together even if both are not ready for the advanced exercises.
- If some of the exercises are still too advanced, substitute exercises from the intermediate workout until you progress.

In This Part

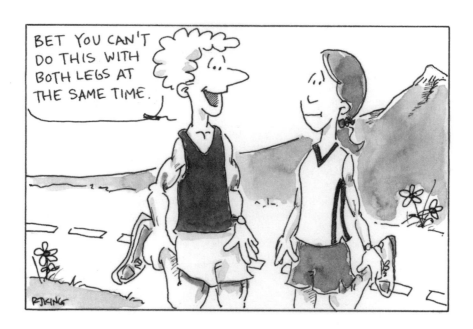

Part 4

Stretch Your Limits

Blessed are the flexible, for they shall not be bent out of shape.

—Unknown

A good morning stretch is quite possibly the best antidote to the worst virus in the world: getting out of bed. That good morning stretch is the difference between pulling the covers over your head and greeting the new day with a smile. You can almost feel the beauty of that stretch right now. Go ahead and give it a try. Don't worry if it's not morning. It works all day long.

See, we know how good stretching feels. So why do we always put it at the bottom of our fitness totem pole? We spend so much time on the exercises that make us *look* good, like cardiovascular exercise and strength training, and so little time on the exercises that actually make us *feel* good.

It's time to move stretching to the top of the list. It's time to make it the Cinderella of our workout program instead of the red-headed stepchild. It's time to stretch early and stretch often and stretch until we can't stretch anymore.

In This Chapter

- ◆ Why stretching is essential to a balanced exercise program

- ◆ How stretching will improve your fitness routine

- ◆ Overstretching and injury

- ◆ When to take a stretch break

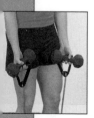
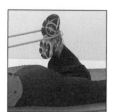
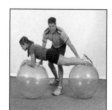
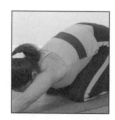
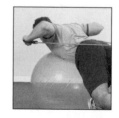
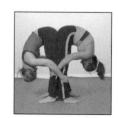

Chapter 16

Stretch It Out

Stretching is probably the most overlooked aspect of any fitness program. If you are one of those people who thinks stretching is not vital to your exercise routine, you are making a huge mistake. Stretching may actually be the most important aspect of your fitness routine, especially as you age. So before you forego the stretching for ten more minutes of aerobics or weight training, read this chapter.

Why Stretch?

Too many people make stretching an afterthought in their exercise routine. They only do it if they have an extra couple minutes at the end of their workout. They only do it if they are really sore from a previous workout. They only do it if they are killing time while they wait for someone to get off their favorite treadmill at the gym. Mistake, mistake, mistake. Remove "only" from those statements and replace it with "always." Stretching should *always* be a part of your exercise routine.

What's all the hype about stretching and what can it do for you and your partner? Well, to answer that, let's take a look at the benefits that regular exercise can have on your muscles.

Don't Sweat It

Too often people skip the stretching part of their workouts because they can't physically see the results it produces. Just because the results of aerobics and weight training are more obvious in the mirror doesn't mean they are more significant than the results you can achieve with a good stretching program. Remember: Fitness goes below the surface of the skin and beyond what the mirror and scale can tell you.

Reduce Muscle Soreness

We've preached enough in this book already about muscle soreness and how it is a common and welcomed part of your exercise routine. We've told you it is your body's response to the muscle damage that occurs as you exercise; that muscle soreness should be expected no matter what your fitness level and that it is a sign, in most circumstances, that you are working hard enough; that you and your partner may experience muscle soreness at different times and from different exercises but that soreness is a necessary part of your exercise routine.

However all of those positive outcomes of muscle soreness don't change the fact that muscle soreness doesn't really feel that great, does it? Muscle soreness is annoying at best and debilitating at worst and at some point you and your partner have probably experienced both ends of the spectrum. As a matter of fact, muscle soreness has probably been the reason that you've cancelled at least one exercise session with your partner, isn't it?

If you or your partner can relate to that scenario, ask yourself: Did you spend at least ten minutes stretching after that workout that caused all of the soreness? Chances are, you didn't. You probably finished the workout and dragged yourself into the shower thinking that the hot water beating down on you would

massage away your pain. Not likely. And before we mislead you, not even stretching will take away all of the muscle pain. The only thing that can cure muscle soreness entirely is rest and recovery and a couple of anti-inflammatory drugs if you are so inclined. But stretching can help to minimize the effects of muscle soreness and leave you feeling only mild discomfort as opposed to crippling pain the next day.

Reduce Risk of Injury

It's no secret that you can actually get injured while working out. There's the danger of dropping a weight on your big toe, tripping while running, or getting hit by a car while you ride your bicycle (just to name a few unlikely incidences). However did you know that the act of actually exercising can hurt you as well?

We probably shouldn't even be telling you this. After all, you don't need another excuse to quit your exercise program before it ever really gets started! But the fact is that muscles shorten over time, and repeated usage, as with exercise, can lead to muscle imbalances in the body. Muscle imbalances can lead to ligament stress and joint damage, which can lead to a long list of other physical issues. But don't dismay. Stretching to the rescue!

The goal of any proper stretching program is to return the muscle to its original resting length. If you can do this, you can ward off almost all of the potential for muscle imbalance to develop in your body. So instead of walking crooked and hunched, you can stand tall and walk proud!

Increase Flexibility

Stand up right now. Bend down and touch your toes. Can you do it? If you can, great! You're off to a good start. If you can't, then you need a stretching program in a bad way.

Increasing your flexibility is not just about being able to touch your toes. It's about being able to bend down and pick your children up and not strain your back in the process. It's about being able to reach for something on a high shelf and not pull a muscle on the way back down. Flexibility is about improving your mobility and *functional fitness.*

> **Training Notes**
>
> **Functional fitness** is the body's ability to more easily perform the activities of daily living. It's a new buzzword in the exercise industry. A lot of exercise training is now geared toward functional fitness instead of simply improving physical appearance.

Increasing your flexibility may not seem so important to you now. Maybe you are young, loose, and limber and don't have a problem with bending, reaching or lifting. However flexibility does tend to decrease as you age. Elasticity in the tissues surrounding the muscles is lost during the aging process and if you weren't working to improve your flexibility in your younger years, you will pay for it when you're older. So before you skip on your stretches, fast-forward a few years to when you're a grandparent. You'll want to be able to pick those grandchildren of yours up with ease.

Stretch = Strength

Strength and stretching go hand and hand. In order to achieve maximum results from your strength-training program, you need to partner it with an equally effective stretching program. Judy Atler, in her book *Stretch and Strengthen*, says, "Strengthen what you stretch, and stretch after you strengthen!" This is a simple rule for creating a balanced exercise program, but why is it necessary?

Think of your muscle like a sausage. (Gross, yes, but go with it.) Your muscle is the sausage and the casing around the sausage is something known as *fascia.* Now if you're the butcher, you can only put so much sausage inside of that casing before it's full, right? No matter how hard you try, you won't get any more inside than what that casing will allow. The same theory applies to your muscles. You can't increase their size any more than what the surrounding fascia will allow. You can train as hard as you would like, but the connective tissue around the muscle is constricting the muscle inside.

> **Training Notes**
>
> **Fascia** is the tough connective tissue that surrounds and protects the muscles in the body. It is also responsible for keeping the muscle in its proper place in the body.

Once again, stretching to the rescue! If you could stretch the sausage casing, you would have room to squeeze more sausage inside, wouldn't you? So if you could stretch the fascia, wouldn't you have more room to grow the muscle inside? Sounds simple enough, right? But stretching the fascia is challenging and it takes work. The best time to attempt this type of stretching is after your workout, when the muscles are full of blood. This will place the most pressure on the fascia and encourage it to stretch.

Stretch Basics

So now you know *why* you should stretch. But *how* should you stretch? Follow these simple rules:

◆ **Stretch both sides of the body equally.** In order to maintain muscle balance, you have to perform equal stretching on both sides. If you are stretching one side more than the other, you are actually doing more harm than good.

◆ **Stretch until you feel tension or pulling, never pain.** In most cases, stretching should feel good. If you are experiencing pain or real discomfort, lighten up.

Workout Worries

Sharp pain during stretching is your body's way of telling you that something is wrong. Don't ignore it. Stop the stretch immediately. Let the muscle relax for a moment and see if the pain dissipates. If you feel any discomfort after you have stopped stretching, you may have pulled the muscle.

◆ **No bouncing!** Bouncing during stretching was once common. The belief was that the bouncing action would cause you to stretch further. However the opposite is actually true. Bouncing activates the body's *stretch reflex*, the mechanism in the body designed to prevent overstretching of the muscles. By engaging in a slow, static stretch, you can bypass the muscle's stretch reflex and allow greater lengthening of the muscle.

Training Notes

The **stretch reflex** is a neuromuscular action in the body which takes place when a muscle is rapidly stretched. When a muscle is abruptly stretched, the brain sends a signal to that muscle to immediately contract. This prevents the muscle from being overstretched. This is a safety mechanism in the body to help prevent injury.

◆ **Breathe!** Most people don't find stretching to be very comfortable. As a result, they hold their breath. However holding your breath prevents an effective stretch. To maximize the stretch, breathe into it. Inhale, and as you exhale, move deeper into the stretch. Continue the breathing, and every time you exhale, sink further into the stretch.

◆ **Hold it.** Many people make the mistake of holding the stretch for only a few seconds. That's not long enough to achieve any of the benefits we discussed earlier in this chapter. To really reap the benefits of the stretch, you should hold it for thirty to sixty seconds. This is long enough for the muscle to relax and lengthen.

◆ **If you strengthened it, stretch it!** There is a stretch for every major muscle group in the body. Do it. Skipping out on some muscle groups will lead to imbalances in your finely toned body. Don't cheat yourself. Stretch it all out.

These rules are only guidelines for your stretching experience. Listen to your body, hold stretches longer if you need to and stretch more often if your body is asking for it.

Stretch Before, Stretch After

The fitness industry is full of debated issues, and this is one of them. It was widely believed that stretching before your workout produced the most positive benefits for your muscles. It was thought that this practice would prepare the muscle for the exercise and help to prevent injury when the more rigorous activity began. Then a bunch of fitness types started doing studies and discovered that stretching before you exercised didn't actually do as much as they once thought. The reason is simple. If you stretched a cold muscle, one that hadn't been warmed up from aerobic activity, it wouldn't really stretch at all. So there went that theory out the window.

Workout Worries

Never stretch a cold muscle. There is absolutely no benefit to this practice but it is a mistake that many exercisers make. Stretching a muscle that hasn't been warmed up can lead to injury because you're forcing that muscle to stretch when its elasticity is at its lowest point.

That's not to say that stretching before you exercise is a bad idea. You just have to do a complete thermal warm-up first. This would include about ten minutes of aerobic activity, involving the large muscle groups. Then after this warm-up, you would spend about ten to fifteen minutes stretching the muscles. The purpose of this short stretching session would mostly be to prevent injury. In this time, you would cool down slightly, so you'd have to warm-up again, and then begin your cardio workout. But are you going to do all that just to get a stretch? We're doubtful.

The post-workout stretch is really the most effective for guaranteeing positive results. After a workout, your muscles are at their warmest and most flexible. At this point, you can get the muscle to relax and encourage its return to the normal resting length. Stretching after your workout will also aid in the removal of the waste products that build in the muscle during an exercise session. Left in the muscles, these waste products can lead to muscle soreness and stiffness. If you only stretched before your workout, you would never reap the benefits of waste product removal and would most likely experience soreness after every workout. That's no fun either.

So what's the best plan for your stretching routine? Well, it's a little bit of both. If you had time during each exercise session, stretching before your workout, after a thermal warm-up, and also after your exercise session would be best. This would guarantee the maximum benefits from your stretching routine. But since you probably won't do this, nor will you have time during every workout, focus on the stretches after your workout if you want to achieve greater flexibility and reduce your risk of getting injured.

Take a Stretch Break

Here are some ways you can squeeze a stretch break into every day:

◆ **In the shower or bath tub.** A great way to start the day on the right foot. The hot water will elevate your muscle temperature just enough to make stretching safe and effective. After your shower or bath, spend some time doing some basic stretches.

◆ **At your desk.** Office stretch breaks are an excellent way to prevent the common workplace injuries that occur from sitting at your desk, in the same position all day long. Try this: Get up from your desk and climb a few flights of stairs to get your muscles warm. When you get back to your desk, do a few stretches for the legs and arms. You might get some funny looks from your co-workers but you'll definitely feel better at the end of the day.

◆ **Waiting in line.** The average person spends way too many hours a week standing in line in various places, grocery stores and post offices among the worst. Don't let this valuable time go to waste. You can do simple neck and hand stretches to alleviate some of the stress and tension that waiting in line can produce. If nothing else, it will keep your hands occupied so you don't strangle the person in front of you who took forty-five grocery items to the express lane!

◆ **In your car.** It seems like traffic is a problem everywhere you go now. Don't let road rage get the best of you. Stretching in the car can not only take your mind off the fact that you've only gone half a mile in the last thirty minutes, but it can also help keep your muscles long and limber. So next time the Sunday drivers are leading the pack, sit back, relax, and stretch!

It's important that you and your partner encourage each other to stretch. It will be tempting at the end of your workout to part ways without doing a complete stretch. Try to make it a mandatory part of every workout. Use the stretching time to plan your next workout or catch up on the other stories you couldn't tell while you were huffing and puffing. Chatter is absolutely acceptable during the stretching portion of your workout, as long as you can breathe at the same time.

Elastic Man: Stretching Too Thin

Of course, with the good comes the bad. As we've already mentioned, the purpose of a stretching routine is to increase the mobility of a joint. However there is a fine line between being mobile and being too mobile. Too much flexibility will cause the joint to become unstable, which can lead to injury. We had to go and complicate things, didn't we?

Before you get all worried that you're a candidate for overstretching, chances are you're not. This problem is usually prevalent in dancers and yoga fanatics who have spent a lifetime working on their flexibility. But you should know it is remotely possible. Here are some of the warning signs:

◆ Pain after stretching

◆ "Popping" sounds in the joints

◆ Arthritis-type aches in the joints

◆ Frequent muscle strains or ligament sprains

◆ Frequent dislocations of any of the joints

If any of these apply to you, back off the stretching and focus on strengthening the weakened joints.

The Least You Need to Know

- Stretching is often overlooked, but is one of the most important aspects of any proper exercise regimen.
- Stretching not only improves the elasticity of the muscle but can also lead to increased muscle development.
- Taking frequent stretch breaks throughout the day can lead to significant improvements in your flexibility.
- Overstretching is just as dangerous as under-stretching when it comes to joint stability.

In This Chapter

- ◆ Why partner stretching is more effective than stretching alone

- ◆ The importance of communication between you and your partner

- ◆ Techniques for effective partner stretching

- ◆ Stretches for every muscle group in the body

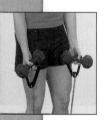
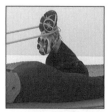
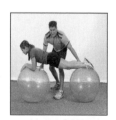
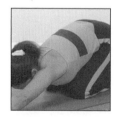
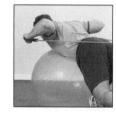
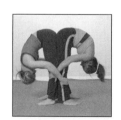

Chapter 17

Partner Stretching

The rack: In ancient times it was used as a torture device. If you were convicted of a crime, you were put on the rack and slowly stretched from hands to feet. Every muscle from fingers to toes would be pulled until the subject cried out in pain. Sounds awful, right?

But eliminate the pain factor and the idea of the rack doesn't sound half bad. Haven't you ever just needed a really good stretch from the top of your head to the bottom of your feet? And no matter how hard you try, you just can't seem to get that complete release of a full body stretch. The idea of getting on a rack and being pulled from one end to the other doesn't sound like torture, it sounds like heaven, doesn't it? Well, we don't think there is a large commercial market for the rack in the twenty-first century, but you've got the next best thing: Your fitness partner! That's right, your trusty sidekick can help you to stretch in such a way that you will feel like you just spent ten minutes on that torture device, without the pain or criminal record.

In this chapter, we'll walk you through the ins and outs of partner stretching. We'll teach you how to safely stretch each other to produce the maximum benefit for your muscles and we'll illustrate partner stretches for every major muscle group in the body.

The Extra Inch

Way, way back in Chapter 4, we talked about the overload principle as it relates to exercise. Well, the same theory applies to stretching. If you stretch only to the point that you can actually reach, you will never make it past the sticking point. If you bend down to touch your toes and you can only reach your knees, how will you ever get to your toes? We'll tell you how. You need a partner push.

Partner-assisted stretching is your secret weapon. By having your partner help you with your stretching program, you will be able to reach that extra inch beyond your sticking point. The one little inch will become several inches over time and soon you will be seeing your toes quite clearly. For some of you, that might be a scary thing, but nothing a pedicure can't fix!

Fit Facts

In order to increase your flexibility, you have to slowly push past your stretch limit to relax and elongate the muscle. This is often hard to do by yourself because you can only reach as far as you can reach. Having a partner to give you the extra, gentle push allows your muscle to stretch to its potential, and over time this helps to increase your range of motion.

If you consider yourself to be very inflexible, this extra inch might take a while to achieve. But rest assured you'll get there faster with a partner than doing it alone.

Partner Stretching Techniques

Before you throw your partner's leg up on your shoulder and push their knee to their nose, you'll want to familiarize yourself with some partner stretching techniques. Assisting your partner with stretching is a serious task and we want to make sure you are prepared. Incorrect stretching could get one or both of you injured. Read this section thoroughly and seek the advice of a personal trainer if you still are unsure.

Workout Worries

Partner stretching is delicate stuff. It would be a good idea to get some proper coaching from a certified personal trainer if you are uncertain about the stretching techniques described here.

Passive Stretching

As the name implies, *passive stretching* is stretching that is initiated by an outside force. In some instances, that outside force could be a piece of furniture, a bar, or the floor. In your case, that outside force is your partner.

The technique for passive stretching is pretty simple:

- Have your partner assume the stretching position.
- Assist the stretching partner by gently pushing them deeper into the stretch (specific instructions for where to spot your partner with particular stretches can be found later in this chapter).
- Encourage your partner to breathe through the stretch.
- Each time your partner exhales, push them further into the stretch.

Training Notes
Passive stretching is stretching that is assisted by an outside force.

The danger with passive stretching is that you, as the assisting partner, are not able to feel the comfort level of your partner. Therefore, you must rely on communication with your partner to determine when you have gone far enough. You can't be the judge of his or her stretch limits, so don't try. Listen to your partner and respect his or her limitations.

PNF

PNF stands for Proprioceptive Neuromuscular Facilitation. Sounds fancy, huh? That's a jazzed-up term for what is really only the contracting and relaxing of a muscle during a stretch. This particular type of stretching is commonly used in physical therapy settings to help facilitate a deeper stretch for patients rehabilitating from injuries. The belief is that fatiguing a muscle during the contraction phase will help it to relax and stretch further in the relaxation phase. PNF stretching is a little more involved than passive stretching. Here's how it works:

◆ Your partner assumes the stretching position.

◆ You, the assisting partner, position yourself to spot the stretcher.

◆ With you providing resistance, the stretching partner contracts the muscle group being stretched and pushes against the resistance.

◆ The stretching partner holds this contraction for about five seconds.

◆ Immediately after your partner releases the contraction, you gently slide your partner into the stretch.

◆ You can repeat the contraction and relaxation several times to encourage a deeper stretch.

PNF is an effective form of stretching, but it should be practiced with caution. You should stay away from PNF if you or your partner have high blood pressure or coronary artery disease because the increased pressure during the contraction phase of the stretch can cause complications with these two conditions. In addition, the contraction phase of the exercise can be uncomfortable for some people. It's best to listen to your partner and do what works for them.

Combining either of these two partner-stretching techniques with some stretching on your own is the best combination for achieving maximum flexibility. The reason is this: While partner stretching will help you to achieve a greater stretch, your muscle will not retain the memory of that stretch because it didn't facilitate it on its own. So after you do some partner stretching, do those stretches again on your own so your muscle has time to remember the movement. This will guarantee greater improvements in your flexibility over time.

Tools of the Trade

When you stretch with a partner, the only tool you really need is your partner. They will be doing most of the work for you. But for the times when you stretch on your own, you may want to have one of these tools handy. Most of these items can be found in your house already.

◆ **Belt or strap.** You can really use a regular belt from your closet. A belt or strap comes in handy when you do stretches that require you to hold on to a body part that you may not be able to comfortably reach yet. You can use it to hold on to that body part and not have to compromise proper form during the stretch. If you don't have a belt, a bath towel will work just fine.

◆ **Stability Ball.** You can use your stability ball that you purchased for your weight-training workouts for stretch training as well.

◆ **Mat.** Break out that exercise mat again. It's best to do your stretches on a softer surface to protect your back. If your mat is not handy, your trusty towel will also work.

Tools that you *will not* need include all of those fancy stretch trainers advertised on late night infomercials. You can do without the high-tech gadgetry and still get a great stretch. Save your money for something worthwhile.

The Partner Stretch Workout

The stretching workout includes stretches for every major muscle group in the body. You can do them all, or you can pick out the ones that coincide with the muscles you trained during your workout. If you choose to use the PNF technique, remember to hold the contraction for five seconds before moving into the relaxation phase. Also remember that it's best to do these stretches with your partner and then on your own so your muscle will better retain the memory of the stretch.

Supine Hamstring Stretch

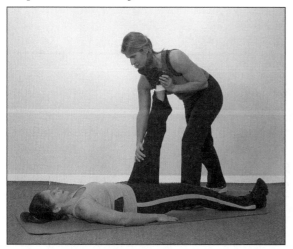

Assisted.

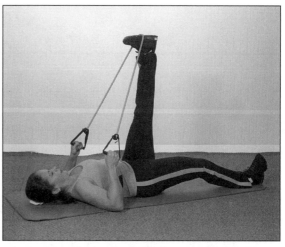

Unassisted.

This is a traditional stretch for the hamstring muscle on the back of the upper leg. The hamstrings are a notoriously tight muscle for most people and the cause of most lower back problems. To insure muscle balance, make sure to perform this stretch equally on both sides of the body. While this exercise can be done with both legs at the same time, we recommend you do it one leg at a time to get the best stretch. If you do this stretch on your own, use your belt or towel for assistance.

Position of Stretcher

◆ The stretcher begins by lying on the floor with one leg extended straight out on the floor and one leg in the air.

◆ The leg in the air should be straight, with no bend in the knee.

◆ Arms can rest comfortably at your sides.

Position of Spotter

◆ The spotter positions himself behind the stretcher's raised leg.

◆ Place one hand on the heel of the stretcher's leg and one hand on the front portion of the thigh, just above the knee, to keep the leg straight.

Movement and Safety Cues

◆ Apply gentle pressure, pushing the stretcher's leg toward his chest.

◆ Be careful not to hyperextend the knee by placing too much force on the knee to keep it straight.

◆ Encourage the stretcher to keep the leg on the floor anchored down so it does not rotate and the pelvis doesn't shift.

Prone Quadriceps Stretch

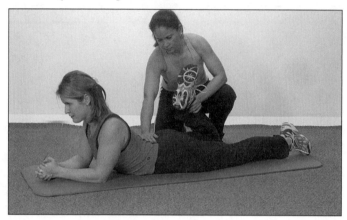

Assisted.

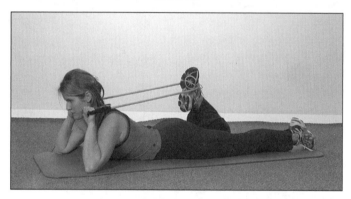

Unassisted.

This stretch is most commonly performed while standing; however it is more easily assisted by a partner when lying in a prone position on the floor. If you are performing this stretch on your own, use your belt or strap for assistance.

Position of Stretcher

- Begin by lying face down, eyes focused on the floor so neck isn't compromised.
- One leg is extended straight out on the floor and the other leg is flexed at the knee with the foot in the air.
- Arms are resting comfortably at your sides.

Position of Spotter

- Place one hand on the stretcher's lower back just above the sacrum (tailbone region).
- Place the other hand on the front part of the stretcher's ankle.

Movement and Safety Cues

- As the stretcher flexes the knee, assist by pushing the foot toward the gluteals.
- Instruct the stretcher to keep her hips anchored in to the floor.
- When stretching, the knee and quadriceps should lift slightly off the ground.

Crossed Leg Rotational Stretch

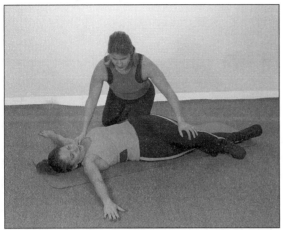

Assisted.

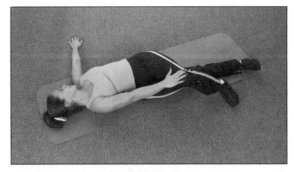

Unassisted.

This is a great stretch for not only the hips and gluteals, but the core muscles as well. However this stretch is not well suited for anyone with lower back pain or vertebrae problems. If you are doing this stretch alone, use the opposite hand to gently pull the top knee across the body.

Position of Stretcher

- ◆ Start by lying supine on the floor with arms extended out to the sides.
- ◆ Extend one leg straight out on the floor.
- ◆ Cross the other leg over top of the straight leg with the knee bent.

Position of Spotter

- ◆ Kneel alongside of the stretcher on the bent leg side.

- ◆ Place one hand on the stretcher's closest shoulder.
- ◆ Place the other hand on top of the knee of the stretcher's bent leg.

Movement and Safety Cues

- ◆ Gently push the knee down to the floor and keep the shoulder down with the other hand.
- ◆ Encourage the stretcher to keep both shoulders in contact with the floor throughout the duration of the stretch.
- ◆ Avoid pinning the knee to the floor. This can cause too much rotation of the spine.

Calf Stretch

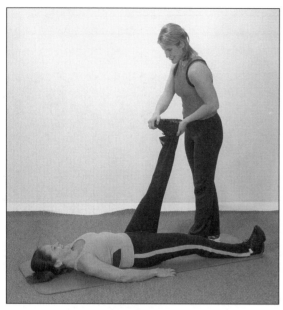

Assisted.

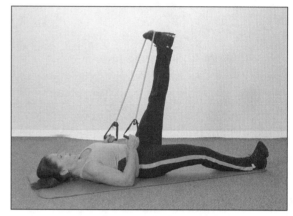

Unassisted.

This stretch focuses on the calf muscle in the lower leg. Walking and running can cause tightening of the calf muscle, which can lead to Achilles' tendon injuries, so be sure to do this stretch often. If you are doing this stretch on your own, use your belt or towel on increase the range of motion at the ankle.

Position of Stretcher

- The stretcher begins by lying on the floor with one leg extended straight out on the floor and one leg in the air.
- The leg in the air should be straight, with no bend in the knee.
- Arms can rest comfortably at your sides.

Position of Spotter

- The spotter positions himself behind the stretcher's raised leg.
- Place one hand on the ball of the stretcher's raised foot as the other hand lifts from the back of the stretcher's heel.

Movement and Safety Cues

- Apply gentle pressure to the ball of the foot, pushing the stretcher's toes toward her face.
- Encourage the stretcher to flex their foot as much as they can on their own to initiate the stretch.
- Instruct the stretcher to push their heel to the ceiling to get the maximum stretch in the calf.

Adductor Stretch

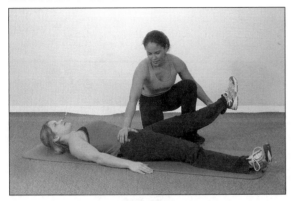

Assisted.

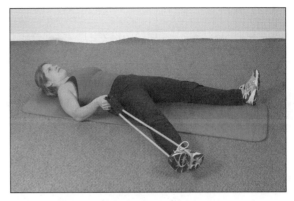

Unassisted.

The adductor muscles are more commonly referred to as the inner thighs. There are many variations of this stretch, the most common being the seated butterfly stretch. This adductor stretch will be performed in a lying position so that one leg can be stretched at a time. If you are performing this stretch alone, use your belt to assist you.

Position of Stretcher

◆ Begin by lying on the floor with both legs extended straight out and arms resting comfortably at your sides.

◆ As you move through the stretch, keep both shoulders in contact with the floor.

◆ Slightly raise one leg off the floor.

Position of Spotter

◆ Kneel next to the stretcher on the raised leg side.

◆ Place one hand on the raised leg of the stretcher, midway between the knee and ankle.

◆ Place the other hand on the lateral side of the opposite hip of the stretcher.

Movement and Safety Cues

◆ Gently pull the raised leg of the stretcher laterally out to the side.

◆ Maintain hip stability by gently pushing on the opposite hip of the stretcher.

◆ Instruct the stretcher to flex the foot of the raised leg to maximize the stretch.

Gluteals Stretch

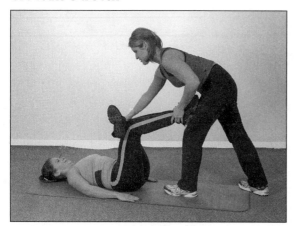

Assisted.

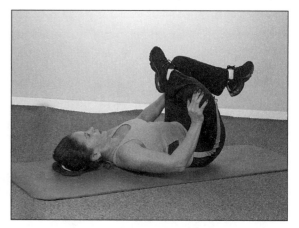

Unassisted.

This is a deep gluteal stretch that will feel great after a leg workout that involves squats or lunges. Remember to stretch each side equally to maintain muscular balance on both sides of the body. If you are doing this stretch alone, you don't need any tools. You can use your arms to assist with the stretch.

Position of Stretcher

◆ Begin by lying supine on the floor with knees bent and feet flat on the floor.

◆ Cross one leg over the other, placing the ankle of the crossed leg just below the knee of the bent leg.

◆ Lift the bent leg off the floor, flexing that hip 90 degrees.

Position of Spotter

◆ Position yourself in front of the exerciser so that the stretcher's foot is against your leg.

◆ Place one hand on the top knee of the stretcher.

Movement and Safety Cues

◆ Using the hand that is on the knee, gently pull that knee toward you as you push the stretcher's opposite knee toward her chest.

◆ Instruct the stretcher to keep her lower back pressed gently in to the floor so the hips don't lift.

◆ Use your leg to lean in to the stretcher to maximize the stretch through the gluteals.

Stability Ball Chest Stretch

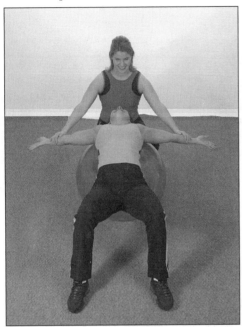

Assisted.

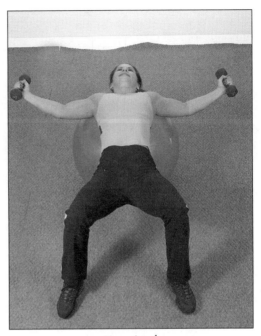

Unassisted.

This stretch is designed to stretch the muscles of the chest and anterior portions of the shoulder. You will get the best range of motion if you do this stretch on a ball, but if you don't have one handy, doing it on a bench will work just as well. If you are doing this on your own, you can get a greater stretch by holding dumbbells in each hand.

Position of Stretcher

◆ Begin seated on the ball and roll into a supine position with your back properly supported on the ball.

◆ Stretch your arms out to the sides with your palms facing toward the ceiling.

◆ Make sure you head is resting on the ball to protect your neck during the stretch.

Position of Spotter

◆ Kneel behind the stretcher's head.

◆ Place your hands on the stretcher's wrist.

Movement and Safety Cues

◆ Apply gentle downward pressure to the stretcher's wrists.

◆ Be careful not to hyperextend the stretcher's elbow. To prevent this, the stretcher should keep a slight bend in her elbow throughout the duration of the stretch.

◆ The stretcher should feel the stretch throughout the chest and shoulder area.

Shoulder Stretch

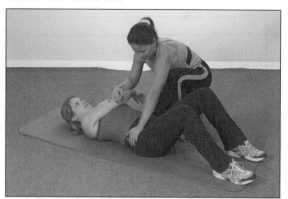

Assisted.

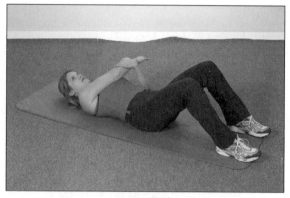

Unassisted.

This shoulder stretch can be performed seated or lying down. This particular stretch concentrates on the rear portion of the deltoid muscle. If you are doing this stretch by yourself, you can use your opposite arm for assistance.

Position of Stretcher

◆ Begin by lying supine on the floor with your knees bent and feet placed flat on the floor.

◆ Place one arm alongside of your body and raise the other arm into the air.

Position of Spotter

◆ Position yourself kneeling next to the stretcher on the opposite side of the raised arm.

◆ Place one hand on the lateral side of the opposite hip of the stretcher.

◆ Place the other hand on the back of the stretcher's raised arm, just below the elbow.

Movement and Safety Cues

◆ While holding on to the stretcher's hip, gently pull the stretcher's arm across her body.

◆ Instruct the stretcher to keep her shoulder away from her ear as the arm is stretched.

Triceps Stretch

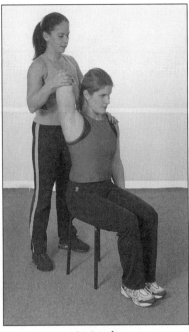

Assisted.

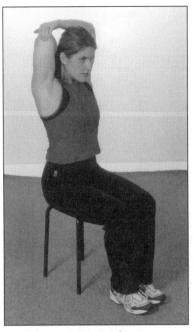

Unassisted.

The triceps are one of the smallest of the major muscle groups in the body and they tend to get sore easily. Spend some time with this triceps stretch to keep the muscle elongated and upper arms from getting too tight. You can do this stretch standing or seated in a chair. If you are doing this stretch on your own, you can use your opposite hand for assistance.

Position of Stretcher

◆ Seat yourself in a chair or on a bench.

◆ With one hand reaching for the end of the bench or chair, raise the other arm up into the air.

◆ Flex the raised arm so that the hand reaches behind your head.

Position of Spotter

◆ Position yourself standing behind the stretcher.

◆ Place one hand on the back of the raised arm just below the elbow.

◆ Place the other hand on the opposite arm midway between the shoulder and elbow.

Movement and Safety Cues

◆ Holding on to the lowered arm for stability, gently push the elbow of the raised arm toward the opposite shoulder.

◆ Instruct the stretcher to keep the spine straight and not to lean into the stretch.

Bicep Stretch

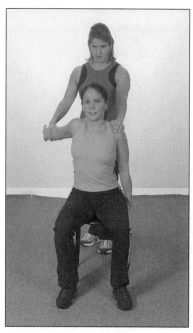

Assisted.

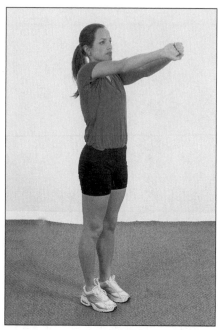

Unassisted.

The bicep can be a hard muscle to effectively stretch. In order to stretch the biceps, the arm must be straight and the wrist must be flexed laterally. If you are doing this stretch by yourself, you can gently pull your fingertips back with your other hand.

Position of Stretcher

◆ Begin by sitting on a bench.

◆ Hold on to the underside of the bench with one hand.

◆ Raise the opposite arm laterally out to the side.

◆ Flex the wrist laterally, reaching the fingertips away from you.

Position of Spotter

◆ Position yourself standing behind the stretcher.

◆ Place one hand behind the shoulder of the resting arm of the spotter. This is the arm that is grabbing the underside of the bench.

◆ Grasp the wrist of the stretcher's extended arm as you gently pull that arm behind the stretcher.

Movement and Safety Cues

◆ As you pull the arm behind the stretcher, push the fingertips towards the stretcher's back.

◆ To keep the torso from twisting with the stretch, stabilize the upper body of the stretcher with your other hand.

◆ Instruct the stretcher to keep the stretching arm as straight as possible.

Seated Upper Back Stretch

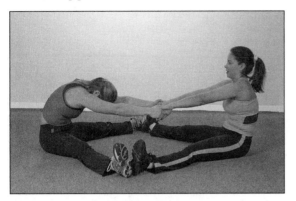

Assisted.

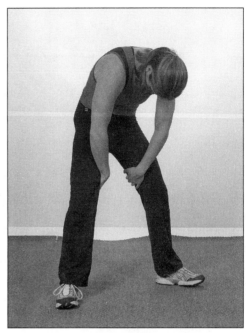

Unassisted.

This is a great stretch for the upper back and latissimus dorsi muscles that will also stretch the hamstrings and lower back region. Both partners can do this stretch at the same time, taking turns being the puller and the stretcher. If you are doing this stretch alone, you can do it standing, holding on to the back of your thighs and lifting your upper back to the ceiling.

Position of Stretcher

- Begin seated on the floor with legs stretched out in front of you about shoulder-width apart.
- Reach both arms out in front of you with palms facing the floor.

Position of Spotter

- Begin seated in the same position as the stretcher.
- Grasp the stretcher's outstretched arms.

Movement and Safety Cues

- Gently pull the stretcher's arms toward your body.
- Instruct the stretcher to round the upper back as you pull.
- Instruct the stretcher to pull away from you as you attempt to pull her toward you.
- Partners can switch roles with the stretcher becoming the spotter and the spotter becoming the stretcher.

Child's Pose Back Stretch

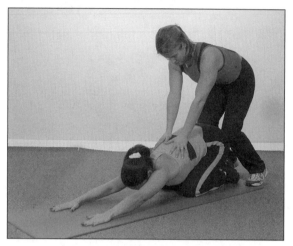

Assisted.

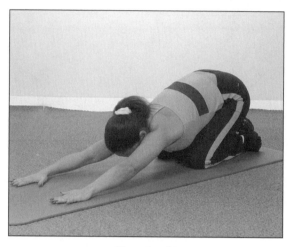

Unassisted.

This stretch is taken from a yoga pose called the child's pose or resting pose. It is a great stretch for the lower back and can also be a great relaxation pose for after a long, hard workout. If you are doing this stretch on your own, there is no assistance needed. Just reach your hands out as far as you can and breathe into the stretch.

Position of Stretcher

- Begin by kneeling on the floor.
- Reach your arms out in front of you and hinge at your hips, lowering your chest to the floor.
- Sit the hips back onto the heels and stretch the arms out as long as they will go.

Position of Spotter

- Position yourself behind the stretcher.
- Place both of your hands on the lower back of the stretcher slightly below the shoulder blades.
- Bend your knees, placing your knees into the stretcher's gluteals.

Movement and Safety Cues

- Using your body weight, gently push your hands into the lower back of the stretcher, pushing her hips closer to her heels.
- Instruct the stretcher to keep the upper body relaxed and the chest sinking in to the floor.

The Least You Need to Know

- Assisted stretching, like that with a partner, can lead to significant gains in flexibility that cannot be achieved alone.
- Stretching with a partner is serious business and can cause injury if done incorrectly.
- Passive and PNF stretching are two common types of partner stretching and both are effective when done properly.
- Stretches should be done with a partner and alone to train the muscle to remember the stretch.

In This Chapter

◆ Why partner yoga will enhance your partner exercise program

◆ How to "yoga breathe" and why it's different from regular breathing

◆ Learning the yoga lingo

◆ Partner yoga poses for the beginner yogi

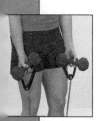
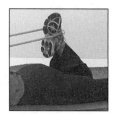
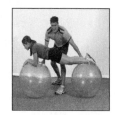
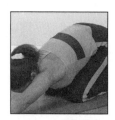
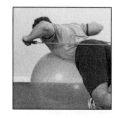
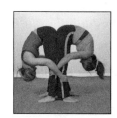

Chapter 18

Yoga-Mania

The fact that you're even reading this chapter is a good sign. It means you're willing to embrace yet another new fitness experience with your partner. Practicing partner yoga will probably be new to both of you and we're glad to be the ones to introduce you to this wonderful fitness practice.

We know it's tempting to skip right to the picture section of this chapter first. You probably want to preview the crazy positions we might have you both in before you commit to reading this whole chapter. But we encourage you to read the chapter first. Try not to form any opinions about yoga or this partner yoga workout until you read everything we have to say about the ancient practice of yoga. We hope to dispel some of the many myths about yoga and encourage you to give it a try with your fitness partner.

So join us as we help you and your partner find your chi.

Finding Your Chi

What is your *chi* and where can you find it? That's a good place to start this yoga discussion. Your chi is not a body part and can't be found in any medical textbooks. Rather, chi refers to a state of consciousness in an individual. It is also commonly referenced as the center of one's being. But what does that really mean? Where is your center, and how can you find it?

Training Notes

Chi, in yoga speak, refers to a vital force in the body that is believed to be inherent in all things. The unimpeded circulation of chi and a balance of negative and positive forms in the body are held to be essential to good health in traditional yoga belief.

Unfortunately, it's not as easy as you think. The practice of yoga is not as cut and dry as with exercise. You see, traditional exercise is goal oriented: How many push-ups can I do? How far can I run? By contrast, yoga is a process where the focus is not on the goal but your own awareness of what you're trying to accomplish. With traditional exercise, you fail if you don't reach your goal. With yoga, you succeed by trying. And that's only part of the beauty of yoga.

The question becomes, can you think outside of your exercise box and embrace this new element of fitness in your program? Can you and your partner commit to try to experience yoga as a process and not as a success or a failure? Can you consider your fitness endeavor outside of pounds and numbers and look for more complete emotional and spiritual health?

For the purpose of this book, finding your chi is about finding your comfort level with this yoga process. We firmly believe that yoga with a partner can be a rewarding experience and can heighten the experience of your fitness relationship. It will be especially significant if both of you are new to the practice of yoga and can learn and develop at the same rate. You will no doubt have some reservations about yoga if you have never done it before, but you and your partner can overcome that apprehension by practicing together.

Take a Deep Breath

With yoga, the breath fuels the exercise and encourages the muscles to relax and deepen the experience of the stretch. We've discussed breathing techniques in several other chapters of this book as a way to encourage a positive muscle response with a particular exercise. However we've really only mentioned that breathing was important, but not how you breathe. With yoga, the actual process of how you breathe is critical to the exercise. Go figure—we had to make this complicated, right?

Before you get discouraged, remember that breathing isn't new to you. You do it all the time, several thousand times a day. So we have a feeling that you will catch on quickly to this. Besides, we're going to give you only the basics of yoga breathing. If you want to learn more, check out *The Complete Idiot's Guide to Yoga.*

To experience a complete, quality yoga breath, try this exercise:

◆ Sit or lie down in a place where you can get comfortable and be relaxed.

◆ Place your hands across your stomach with your fingertips touching over top of your belly button.

◆ Slowly inhale. Breathe through your nose only. The breath should fill the belly, lift the rib cage, and fill the lungs.

- Allow the breath to expand your belly. You should feel your fingertips slowly separate as you continue to inhale.

- As you exhale, contract the abdominals, letting the belly collapse and the fingertips come back together.

- Learn to feel the breath in the sides and the back of the body. Breathing shouldn't reside in the front of your body only.

- Repeat this breath cycle until you feel relaxed.

Don't Sweat It

"Yogis count life not by number of years but number of breaths."

—Swami Vishnudevananda

Yoga breathing is a great practice for stress relief. Before stress buries you, engage in one minute of yoga breathing. It will calm your emotions and regulate the physiological responses to stress including increased heart rate and blood pressure. We mentioned earlier in this book that stress and life can get in the way of your and your partner's best fitness intentions. One minute of yoga breathing can help you both to reconnect and refocus on the importance of your health and the commitment you made to each other way back in Chapter 1.

Up Dog, Down Dog

No, you don't need a dog to perform yoga, although we're sure there is someone out there right now writing a book on yoga for your pet! But Up Dog, Down Dog has nothing to with your pet. It's the name given to two different yoga poses, the Up Dog and the Down Dog. Sounds crazy, right?

These names are actually much simpler than the real *Sanskrit* yoga names that are given to these poses, Urdhva Mukha Svanansana and Adho Mukha Svanasana. Say those ten times fast! Sanskrit is the ancient Hindu language that yoga terminology is derived from. Since most of the terms do not easily translate into English or other Western languages, they are often named for what the pose looks like rather than what the Sanskrit term actually translates to. Here are some common yoga poses along with their Sanskrit and English names.

Yoga Poses

English	Sanskrit
Child's Pose	Garbhasana
Camel	Ushtrasana
Table	Svanasana
Tree	Vrikshasana
Eagle	Garudasana
Cobra	Bhujangasana
Boat	Navasana

Visualize and Energize

A large part of the yoga process is being able to put yourself in a position to open up your energy channels. These energy channels, also called *chakras*, are places from which energy originates in the body. It is believed that when the body is positioned correctly, these channels can open and positive energy can be released to flow through the body. The ability to open your chakras takes time and focus, and you and your partner should not expect to feel this energy flow immediately. However this does not mean that positive things are not taking place in your body. Everything from the simple complete breath to the most difficult yoga pose can evoke healthy responses in your body's systems.

Many people mistake yoga to be only a relaxing and calming form of meditation. On the contrary, many forms of yoga can be extremely energizing and powerful, making them more of a workout than you would imagine. What's more, yoga can actually help you to burn more calories during other types of exercise. How, you ask? Take running. Practicing yoga will help you improve flexibility, strength, and posture, all of which are key for proper running technique. By having better running form, you can become more efficient and burn more calories in less time out on the road, all thanks to yoga!

Visualizing these benefits during your yoga practice will open your mind to all of the possibilities. If you can see yourself getting stronger and more flexible with every pose, you will!

The Partner Yoga Workout

Pairing up for yoga is going to be a lot like pairing up for any of the other workouts in this book. You need to listen to your partner and adjust your workouts according to each other's needs.

In this workout, you use gentle pressure, body weight, and touch to maximize the stretches and encourage alignment throughout all of the postures. This yoga workout will also be different from the other ones illustrated in this book because you will not be focusing on your outward physical feelings of fatigue or tiredness. Instead you focus on the inward feelings of energy and vitality. If at any time you start to feel your concentration fade, watch your partner. You serve as mirrors for each other and this reflection can help you stay on track and keep your focus on the postures and poses.

Let's get started.

Double Moon Pose

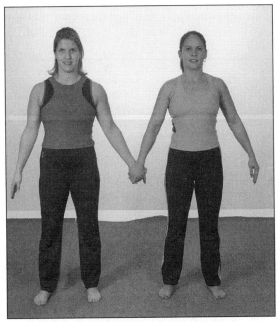

Pose One.

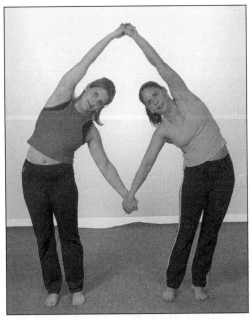

Pose Two.

The Double Moon Pose is a great beginning posture to start your yoga workout. The double moon pose quiets the mind and helps partners to focus on their postures and spinal alignment. This crescent-shaped pose also provides a great side stretch and opens the rib cage for deeper breathing.

Pose One

◆ Partners stand side by side with their inside feet about 3 feet apart.

◆ Clasp inside hands together.

◆ Slightly tighten or flex the muscles in the knees, thighs, stomach, and buttocks and distribute your body weight evenly between both feet.

◆ Begin a slow, deep inhale, and on the exhalation, bring the outside arm up overhead.

◆ Keep the spine lengthened as you reach for the ceiling.

Pose Two

◆ Begin a side bend toward your partner.

◆ Your outside hip should push completely away from your partner as you bring your hands together over your heads.

◆ Keep the outside shoulder behind your outside ear so that the stretch can be experienced throughout the torso.

◆ Focus the breath into the outside ribs.

◆ Hold this pose for four to six breath cycles.

Double Table Pose

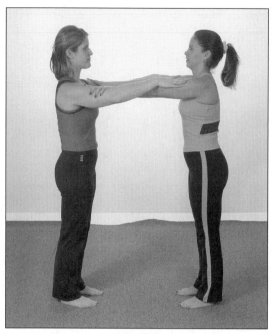

Pose One.

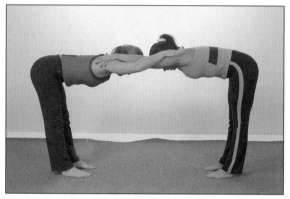

Pose Two.

The Table is a forward-bending pose that focuses on opening the chest and shoulders as well as lengthening the muscles in the back of the legs. This posture is great after long car or plane rides or when you feel the need for a good spine stretch. It also prepares the body for more forward-bending poses.

Pose One

◆ Stand facing your partner with arms outstretched in front of you, parallel to the ground.

◆ Grasp the top of your partner's upper arms with your hands.

◆ Your spine is long and lengthened with your shoulders relaxed and away from your ears.

◆ Slowly bend forward while taking small steps away from your partner.

Pose Two

◆ Lengthen the back of your legs by lifting your buttocks toward the ceiling.

◆ Lengthen the spine by flattening your back and pulling your hips away from your shoulders.

◆ On the exhalation, allow the shoulders to relax and the chest to open.

◆ Hold for four to six breath cycles.

Double Chair

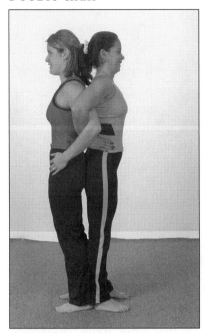

Pose One.

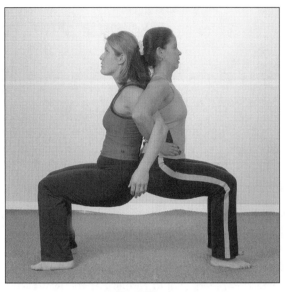

Pose Two.

The Double Chair is a powerful strengthening pose that builds leg strength and encourages good spinal alignment. With this pose, partners have to learn to trust each other and become keenly aware of their partner's balance in order to counterbalance the posture. Partners need good leg development to maintain this posture properly.

Pose One

◆ Begin standing back-to-back with your partner and link arms.

◆ Anchor your lower back and sacrum (tail bone region) to your partner's.

◆ Feet are about hip-width apart and the spine is tall and long.

Pose Two

◆ Begin by consciously pressing your backs against each other and take a few small steps away from each other.

◆ Lean against each other and continue stepping out, sinking your tailbones to the floor as you walk further out.

◆ Stop when you thighs are parallel to the floor.

◆ To keep from sinking to the floor, maintain the resistance on your partner's lower back and distribute the rest of your weight through your heels and into the floor.

◆ Hold for four to six breath cycles.

Double Forward Bend

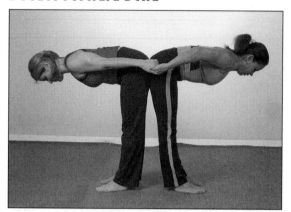

Pose One.

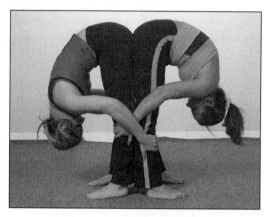

Pose Two.

This Double Forward Bend looks like the exact opposite of the Table. It is also a balance pose that stretches and strengthens the back of the body from the heels through the top of the head. Partners should remember to always move slowly when spinal flexion is involved in the pose. Don't be surprised if you fall forward on your first few attempts. If you feel yourself starting to fall, don't forget to let go of your partner's hands!

Pose One

◆ Begin by standing back-to-back with your partner with your hands linked.

◆ As you inhale, lengthen the spine and lift the top of the head toward the ceiling.

◆ As you exhale, slowly bend forward. It's okay to take small steps away from your partner to maintain your balance.

Pose Two

◆ Allow your chest to collapse completely to your knees.

◆ To enhance the stretch, press your buttocks together by pulling with your hands.

◆ At this point, you can change your hand position, and grasp the back of your partner's calf muscles.

◆ Gently pull your forehead to your knees as you lift your tailbone toward the ceiling.

◆ Hold for four to six breath cycles.

Double Warrior Pose

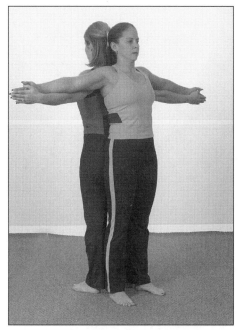

Pose One.

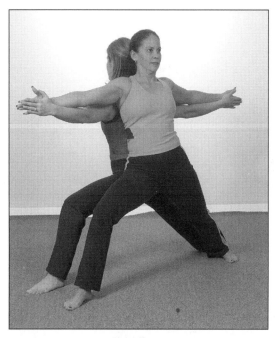

Pose Two.

The Double Warrior pose is a balance pose that strengthens the muscles in the arms and legs and tones the abdominal organs. Named for a fierce warrior, this pose is also designed to increase stamina and invigorate the system. Partners once again must trust each other to maintain balance during this pose.

Pose One

◆ Partners begin by standing back-to-back with their feet about 3½ feet apart.

◆ Both partners should turn one foot out to the side and keep the other foot facing forward. The heel of the out-turned foot should line up with the instep of the foot that is facing forward.

◆ Partners raise their arms to shoulder height and link hands.

◆ Pull toward your partner to form a connection between your upper backs.

Pose Two

◆ As you exhale, bend your front knee so that your thigh is parallel to the floor.

◆ Partners should move into the position at the same time, keeping the connection with their upper backs.

◆ Turn your head toward your bent leg and look out over top of your outstretched arms.

◆ Do not lean forward or backward. Instead sink down into the pose.

◆ Hold for four to six breath cycles.

Double Butterfly

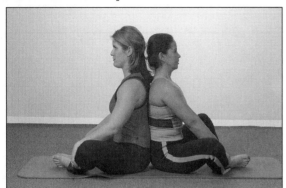

Pose One.

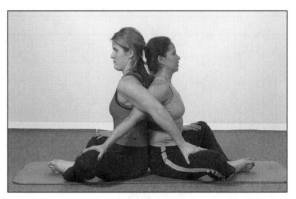

Pose Two.

This is a variation of the very common Butterfly stretch. This yoga posture is a relaxing pose that focuses on opening the hips and aligning the spine. Partners should be aware of each other's limits when pressing each other's knees to the floor. Because you are sitting back-to-back and will not be able to make eye contact during the posture, make sure you vocalize your limit to your partner.

◆ Partners begin sitting on the floor back-to-back.

◆ Bring the soles of your feet together and place them as close as you comfortably can to your body.

◆ Make a connection with your partner's spine by pressing your backs together.

Pose Two

◆ Inhale and reach your hands behind you, placing them on your partner's knees.

◆ Exhale as you gently press your partner's knees toward the floor.

◆ As you continue to breathe, relax the hips, thighs, and ankles.

◆ Hold for four to six breath cycles.

Butterfly Fish

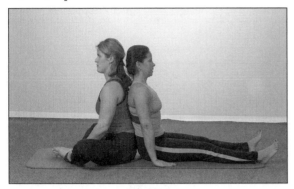

Pose One.

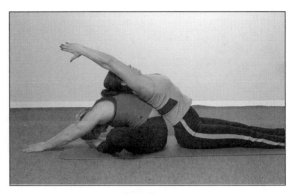

Pose Two.

This posture is a combination of a hip-opening forward bend with a chest-opening backward bend. Once again, partners must communicate their personal limitations with this stretch. For the butterfly partner, the bend begins at the hips. For the fish partner, the bend extends from the lower back.

Pose One

- ◆ Partners begin by sitting on the floor back-to-back.
- ◆ The fish partner extends her legs out in front of her.
- ◆ The butterfly partner brings the soles of her feet together and places them as close as she comfortably can to her body.
- ◆ Partners make a connection with each other's spines by pressing their backs together.
- ◆ Both partners inhale as they lengthen the spine.

Pose Two

- ◆ The butterfly partner exhales and slowly starts to bend forward at the hips. Arms extend out in front of you.
- ◆ The fish partner exhales and slowly moves into a back bend over top of her partner.
- ◆ The fish partner's hands are together in a prayer position with the arms extended overhead.
- ◆ Partners breathe together and relax into the pose.
- ◆ Hold for four to six breath cycles.
- ◆ Change positions and repeat the posture.

Double Boat

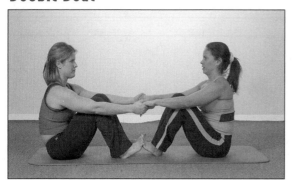

Pose One.

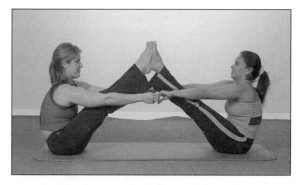

Pose Two.

This posture is a challenging balance posture that requires some abdominal strength and spinal stability. Doing this stretch pose with a partner enhances the stretching of the hamstrings in the back of the legs. Partners can adjust the distance between themselves to find the angle that works best for both of them.

Pose One

◆ Partners begin seated facing each other.

◆ Feet are flat on the floor with toes pointed up to the ceiling.

◆ Partners reach forward and link arms by grasping each other's wrists.

◆ Both partners inhale, lifting the spine and expanding the chest.

Pose Two

◆ On the exhale, partners press against each other's foot and use the resistance to straighten one leg, extending their feet to the ceiling.

◆ Partners can hold in this position until they gain their balance.

◆ Using the same technique, extend the other leg.

◆ As you find your balance, use your arms for support.

◆ Arms should be parallel to the floor as you hold this pose for four to six breath cycles.

Double Spinal Twist

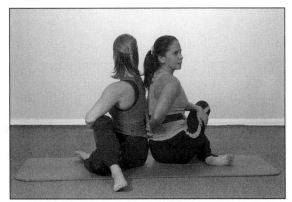

Pose One.

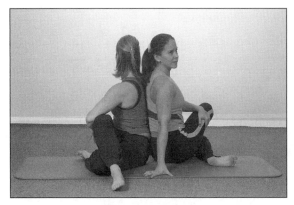

Pose Two.

The Spinal Twist posture is excellent for relieving tension in the lower back and massaging the internal organs. This exercise is not recommended for partners with lower back problems or if one or both partners are pregnant. If you cannot lock arms in the twisting position, simply place your back hand behind you and reach your front hand in front. You can work your way up to the hand lock with practice.

Pose One

◆ Partners begin by sitting side by side, facing in opposite directions.

◆ Both partners bend their inside leg underneath them and cross their outside leg on top of the bottom leg.

◆ The foot of the top leg is pressed flat into the floor.

◆ Both partners initiate a twist away from each other.

Pose Two

◆ Partners connect their opposite hands together so that the front hand of one partner connects with the back hand of the other partner.

◆ Both partners inhale, lengthening the spine.

◆ On the exhale, both partners twist, using their connected arms to pull each other further into the twist.

◆ Hold for four to six breath cycles.

Double Dancer

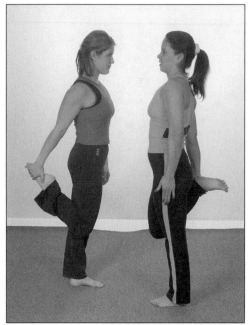

Pose One.

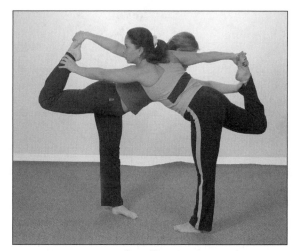

Pose Two.

While dancers require grace, this pose only looks graceful. You don't have to be able to dance at all to complete this posture. It does require balance and some hip and hamstring flexibility to perform. If you have difficulty using your partner as support, practice using the wall first, and then move to holding on to your partner.

Pose One

◆ Partners begin by standing facing each other with their inside shoulders lined up.

◆ Sink your left foot firmly into the ground and lift your right foot behind you, holding your right ankle with your right hand.

◆ Both partners inhale, lengthening their spines and expanding their chests.

Pose Two

◆ As you exhale, lean forward slightly, and reach your left arm straight out.

◆ With your left arm, grasp your partner's right foot.

◆ Inhale again as you lift your right knee and foot toward the ceiling.

◆ Hold for four to six breath cycles.

◆ Switch sides and repeat the posture.

Kneeling Crescent Moon

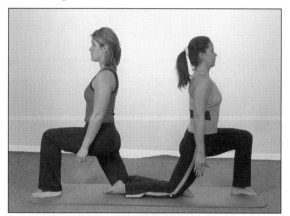

Pose One.

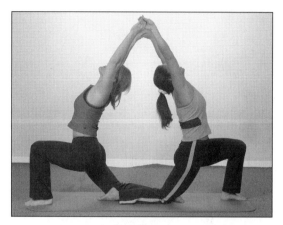

Pose Two.

This pose is a variation on the traditional Crescent Moon, which is done in a standing position. A great stretch for the hips and abdomen, this pose can also be effective in opening the chest and shoulder muscles. As with any back-bending postures, partners should make sure they are warmed up and ready for the challenge. If back problems persist with either partner, skip this pose.

Pose One

- ◆ Partners begin by standing back-to-back.
- ◆ Both partners step their left legs forward, placing their foot on the floor about four feet in front of their left foot.
- ◆ Both partners slowly bring their left knee to the floor, moving into a lunge position.
- ◆ Both partners inhale and sink their hips down into the stretch.
- ◆ On the exhale, partners should push further into the lunge pose.

Pose Two

- ◆ On the next inhale, both partners reach their hands above their heads.
- ◆ As they begin to exhale, both partners lean back, bringing their hands together and reaching their heads back toward each other.
- ◆ Hold for four to six breath cycles.
- ◆ Switch legs and repeat the postures.

Double Triangle

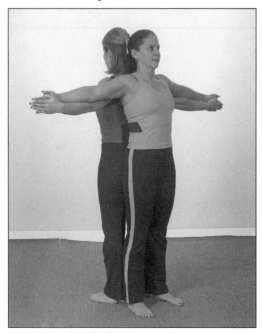

Pose One.

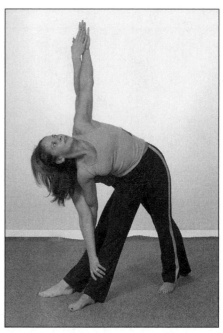

Pose Two.

The Triangle pose engages every part of the body. It strengthens the core, opens the hips and shoulders, and stretches the legs. In traditional yoga, the triangle pose creates a series of triangles, which serves to heat the body and energize the spirit. Doing this posture with a partner will help you maintain proper alignment of the hips and shoulders.

Pose One

- Partners begin standing back-to-back with their feet about 3 or 4 feet apart.
- Both partners extend their arms out to the sides, raising them to shoulder height and intertwining their hands behind each other's arms.
- Both partners pivot one foot so that it points in the direction they are about to bend.

Pose Two

- Both partners inhale and lengthen the spine.
- On the exhale, both partners extend out from their hips and slowly lower their front hand down to their leg as they lift their back hand up to the ceiling.
- Once in this pose, partners can cross their lower hands and support themselves on their partner's lower leg.
- Partners can also cross their upper hands as they reach toward the ceiling.
- Hold for four to six breath cycles.
- Switch to the other side and repeat the posture.

Downward Dog Back Bend

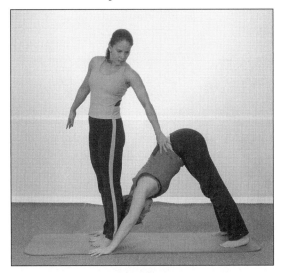

Pose One.

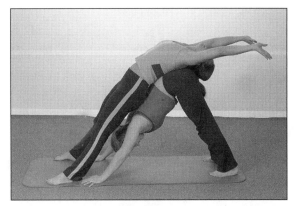

Pose Two.

While backward bends are usually a very advanced move, using your partner's downward dog pose helps to practice this posture safely. The downward dog partner gets a great stretch through the hamstrings and back of the legs while the back-bend partner gets an invigorating chest opener. Back-bending is not recommended for any partner with acute spine or neck injuries.

Pose One

- ◆ Downward dog partner positions himself on his hands and knees with his toes tucked under his feet.
- ◆ While pushing the palms into the floor, extend the legs and lift the hips, moving into an upside down V position.
- ◆ As you push your heels to the floor, lift your seat bones to the ceiling.
- ◆ Back-bend partner stands with her feet between her partner's hands.
- ◆ Using one hand on your partner's back for support, slowly lower your hips down to your partner's back, positioning the buttocks in the middle of your partner's back.

Pose Two

- ◆ Back-bend partner inhales, reaching the arms up over her head.
- ◆ On the exhale, push your hips forward as you arch your back.
- ◆ Your upper back should come in contact with your partner's lower back and sacrum.
- ◆ Hold for four to six breath cycles.
- ◆ Switch roles and repeat the posture.

The Least You Need to Know

- ◆ Yoga breathing can significantly reduce stress and feelings of anxiety.
- ◆ Partner yoga, when performed properly, can increase your calorie-burning capabilities in other areas of your exercise program.
- ◆ The partner yoga workout should be approached with caution, since some of the exercises will be challenging.
- ◆ Since most of the partner yoga poses are mirror images, the yoga poses can be slightly modified if you are doing them alone.

In This Chapter

◆ What Pilates is and why it's so popular

◆ The basic Pilates fitness concepts and how they can enhance your partner workout routine

◆ A Pilates breath and how it's different from yoga and regular breathing

◆ The partner Pilates workout

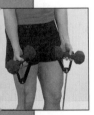
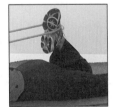
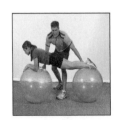
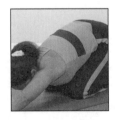
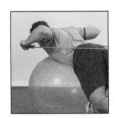
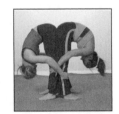

Chapter 19

Partner Pilates

We know you've heard the word before. Pilates is the current buzzword in the fitness industry. It's the Hollywood fitness phenomenon and everyone is doing it. So why aren't you?

In this chapter, we will introduce you and your partner to the Pilates concept, how and where it originated, and why it is so popular in the fitness culture today. We'll teach you how to incorporate some of the basic Pilates concepts into your workouts, and how to safely and effectively coach your partner through the exercises.

Puh-LAH-teez

Now that you're getting trendy with workout lingo, we want to keep you in the loop. So before you go around telling your friends that you're a PI-lates guru, learn how to say the word. It's three syllables, not two, and it's pronounced puh-LAH-teez. Try that out loud.

So what exactly is Pilates and where did it get that crazy name? Pilates is named after its founder and creator, Joseph Pilates, a German immigrant. He developed this form of exercise as a way to combine elements of yoga with the biomechanical operations of the body. Pilates exercises are designed to improve muscle control, flexibility, coordination, strength, and tone by encouraging muscle balance and spinal flexibility. Each exercise is designed to focus on the smaller muscle groups and to maximize the stretch between each vertebrae in the spine. The result: Longer, leaner muscles. Who wouldn't want that?

Well, everyone would, of course. But the question is how do you turn your body into that biomechanical force of nature? How do you create that muscle balance and stretch your spine so much that you finish a Pilates workout feeling two inches taller than when you started?

The answer is: Control. You see, Pilates is all about using the power of your mind to unleash the power of your body.

Don't Sweat It

Joseph Pilates dubbed his revolutionary method of exercise "the art of contrology" because of its emphasis on the mind's control of the body.

If that sounds a little new-agey to you, don't worry, you're not alone. We have fast come to realize that the fitness industry is obsessed with "mind–body" connectivity and Pilates definitely falls into this category. The difference is that Pilates focuses equally on the meditative aspect and the physical aspect. To help understand the concept of Pilates, think of your body as the forklift and your mind as the forklift operator. While the forklift is an awkward piece of equipment to operate (as if we would know), an experienced operator can maneuver that long arm with grace and precision. Pilates is built on the principle that any body can move with the grace of a dancer if they encourage the appropriate muscles. How about that? You and your partner, a graceful duo twirling around the stage. And you thought you were just in this to get a little exercise!

What's In It for You

At this point, we've thrown so many new and wild exercises and fitness concepts at you that you've probably don't even want to think about adding another one to your list. So why should you try this partner Pilates workout with your fitness buddy? Because we said so! But if you need a few more reasons, take a look:

◆ **Rehabilitate from injury.** Have you had a nagging injury, maybe chronic knee or back pain, which has been sticking around for a while? Chances are that Pilates exercises can help. Pilates is popular among injured dancers who use the exercises to pinpoint and correct the source of their pain. Since most chronic injuries develop from muscle imbalances, the Pilates exercises, which focus on creating muscular balance in the body, can help to alleviate your pain.

◆ **Create firm, elongated muscles.** Traditional strength-training exercise tends to focus on the *concentric contraction*, or shortening phase, of the movement. This shortens the muscle and can make it bulky and hard. This is the reason we encourage so much stretching at the end of your workouts—to stretch the muscle back out. However, Pilates exercises are designed to strengthen the muscle during the *eccentric contraction*, or lengthening phase, of the movement. This creates a longer and stronger muscle. So if you're looking for muscle tone without all the bulk, Pilates is a great compliment to your regular strength-training exercise program.

Training Notes

The **concentric contraction** of an exercise refers to the phase of the exercise when the muscle shortens. In most cases, this refers to the flexing part of the movement. During a bicep curl, the concentric contraction occurs when you lift the weight, flexing the elbow.

The **eccentric contraction** of an exercise refers to the phase of the exercise when the muscle lengthens. This is usually the extension part of the movement. During a bicep curl, the eccentric contraction occurs when you lower the weight back down, extending the elbow.

◆ **More for the core!** Pilates exercises are great for strengthening the core muscles of the abdominals and lower back. Most of the exercises involve some sort of stabilization of these muscles to perform movement in other parts of the body. This translates to hard core (excuse the pun) abdominal and lower back strengthening, which means great looking abs and a strong back for you!

◆ **Improve body mechanics.** Wouldn't you feel better if you could move better? Pilates has the potential of giving you the freedom to move with better posture, coordination, and balance. You can enjoy more efficient and graceful movement with the ability to breathe deeper and feel more relaxed. Improving your body mechanics can make a tremendous difference in the quality of your life and your physical appearance. When you feel better, you look better, too!

◆ **Improve posture and alignment.** After a few Pilates sessions, you'll probably start to feel like you are standing a little straighter and walking a little taller. That's because Pilates really focuses on lengthening the spine and creating space between the vertebrae. This may not sound so important to you now, but when you're eighty-five years old and have shrunk to four feet tall, you'll wish you had spent a little time with your Pilates exercises!

Take Another Deep Breath

Here we go, teaching you how to breathe again. Believe it or not, Pilates involves a totally different type of breath, separate even from yoga. While the two are similar, yoga breathing is focused in the belly, and Pilates breathing is focused in the back. Breathing into your back?

How exactly does that work? The best way to understand *posterior lateral rib cage breathing* is to try this exercise with your partner.

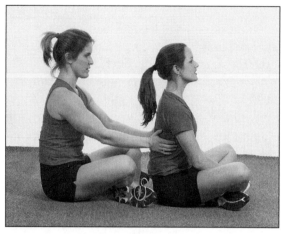

Breathing exercise.

Training Notes

Posterior lateral rib cage breathing is the description given to the Pilates breath. It involves expanding the posterior lateral rib cage portion of the back on the inhale and letting it fall and collapse on the exhale.

◆ Have your partner sit in front of you with her back to you.

◆ Place your hands around the posterior lateral portion of your partner's rib cage.

◆ Gently wrap your fingertips around your partner's rib cage.

◆ Now instruct your partner to inhale. As she inhales, her breath should expand the posterior portion of her rib cage. As she does this, your hands should slightly spread out to the side with your partner's expanding rib cage.

◆ Instruct your partner to inhale without letting the abdomen rise.

♦ As your partner exhales, encourage her to contract the rib cage and pull her pelvic floor up and abdominals down towards the spine.

Reverse roles and let your partner experience the breath by holding on to you. This exercise can give you a greater awareness of what a posterior lateral rib cage breath should feel like.

So why the special breath? Pilates breathing encourages stretching of the muscles between the ribs. This allows for greater mobility in the rib cage. In addition, as you exhale, some of the very hard-to-reach abdominal muscles are activated to engage the pelvic floor. You actually get an abdominal workout just by breathing! You can't beat that!

The Partner Pilates Workout

This Pilates workout is going to be another new and exciting adventure for you and your fitness partner. You will be coaching each other through another challenging set of exercises that will further define your hard-working muscles.

We're assuming that both of you are going to be new to the Pilates workout, so don't take on too much at first. It's tempting to want to maximize the intensity of the exercise when you first get started by doing many repetitions. However, we suggest you do fewer repetitions at the start, and try to focus on the muscle lengthening aspect of the exercise for the first couple of sessions. This will help to encourage the muscle to completely stretch before you tackle the strengthening aspect of the exercises. As you improve, add repetitions and you will really start to reap the benefits of this awesome workout.

The Partner Hundred

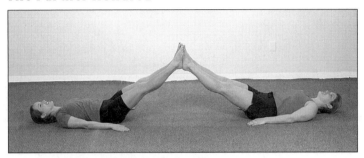

Start/finish.

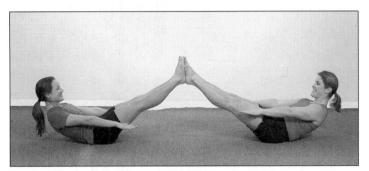

Midpoint.

The exercise gets its name from the number of repetitions that are involved in the exercise. But don't get scared off yet. While you will do one hundred repetitions, it's not as bad as it seems. The hundred is used as part of a warm-up for every Pilates workout. It gets the core warmed up and ready to go. It is also a great exercise for increasing abdominal strength. Just try it!

Position of Exercisers

Note that both partners exercise at the same time.

◆ Both partners begin by lying supine on the ground, toe to toe.

◆ Slightly raise legs off the ground to a comfortable height, keeping feet pressed against each other's.

◆ Curl head and shoulders off the mat.

◆ With arms extended alongside of their bodies, partners raise arms 6 inches off the ground.

Movement

◆ Without moving the legs, partners pump their arms up and down in time with breathing in to a count of six and breathing out to a count of five.

◆ Partners do this ten times in a row.

◆ Partners can remind each other to keep the neck and shoulders relaxed and the arms and legs strong.

The Partner Roll Up

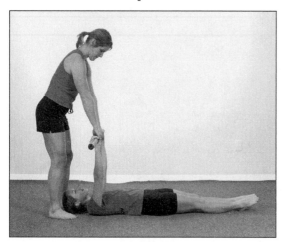

Start/finish.

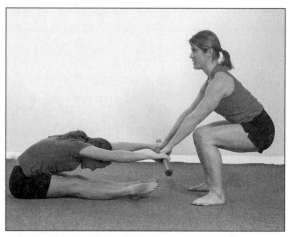

Midpoint.

In this exercise, the partner serves to maximize the stretching movements. It's best to use a stick or bar to assist with this exercise. If one is not available, you can use a rolled up towel. As with any assisted stretching, the exercising partner needs to communicate his or her limits to the spotting partner to avoid injury.

Position of Exerciser

◆ The exerciser begins supine on the floor with legs extended.

◆ Arms are extended up toward the ceiling, holding a straight bar between the hands.

◆ Feet are flexed and rib cage is anchored down into the belly button.

Position of Spotter

◆ The spotter begins by standing at the head of the exerciser, holding on to the same bar.

◆ The spotter will slightly pull on the bar to create a stretch for the exerciser.

Movement

◆ The exerciser begins the roll up, curling her head off the mat and rolling up through the spine to a seated position.

◆ As the exerciser moves, the spotter keeps a resistance on the bar by pulling up toward the ceiling to continue the stretch for the exerciser.

◆ The exerciser stretches all the way forward, reaching the bar out toward the toes.

◆ In this position, the spotter is now at the feet of the exerciser, pulling on the bar to heighten the stretch for the exerciser. The spotter can move into a squat position and get a stretch herself!

◆ The exerciser will reverse the movement, lowering one vertebrae to the floor at a time, and the spotter will return to the starting position.

◆ Repeat six times.

The Partner Spine Stretch

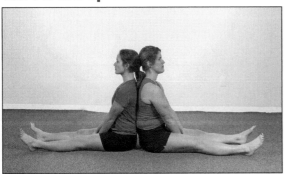

Start/finish.

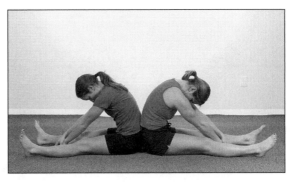

Midpoint.

This spine stretch is one of the most thorough stretches you can do for your spine. As you roll forward, you stretch the spine from the cervical vertebrae at the top of your neck down to the sacrum at your tailbone. The result is an opening of the spaces between the vertebrae and a lengthening of the spine. Do this one early and often!

Position of Exercisers

Note that both partners exercise at the same time.

◆ Exercisers begin seated back-to-back with their legs extended in front of them.

◆ Arms are outstretched in front of their bodies, hands placed on top of each other with fingertips on the floor.

◆ Partners focus on pressing their lower backs together to create a connection of their spines.

Movement

◆ Both partners inhale and sit tall.

◆ As they exhale, partners stretch forward, reaching their hands toward their toes.

◆ Partners keep their lower backs touching as they round the upper back to reach their arms out as far as they will go.

◆ Partners inhale again and round back up to the seated position.

◆ With every repetition partners should feel as though they are sitting taller.

◆ Repeat six to eight times.

Partner Saw

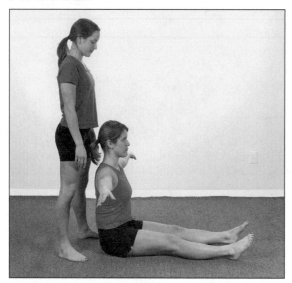

Start/finish.

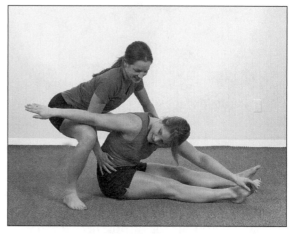

Midpoint.

The saw, a name we can't quite figure out, is another great stretch for lengthening the spine and encouraging spinal rotation. In this exercise, partners assist each other in deepening the stretch and maintaining proper body positioning. The exerciser should focus on keeping both sitz bones (the bones you sit on) in contact with the floor and the hips stabilized as they rotate. This allows for greater lengthening of the spine.

Position of Exerciser

◆ The exerciser begins seated on the floor with legs extended out in front slightly wider than hip width.

◆ Arms are extended out to the sides, slightly in front of the shoulders.

◆ Spine is tall and sitz bones remain in contact with the floor throughout the exercise.

Position of Spotter

◆ The spotter begins by standing behind the exerciser.

◆ Place one hand on the exerciser's right hip and one hand on the exerciser's right shoulder.

◆ Grasp the hip with your hand and hold tightly.

Movement

◆ The exerciser rotates the spine toward the left, reaching the right hand toward the little toe on the left foot.

◆ The spotter stabilizes the exerciser's right hip by gently pulling back to restrict its movement.

◆ As the exerciser reaches forward, the spotter gently pushes on the exerciser's right shoulder to deepen the stretch to the left foot.

◆ The exerciser slowly returns to the starting position.

◆ Repeat eight times on each side.

Partner Teaser

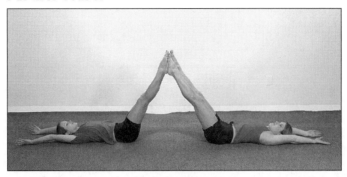

Start/finish.

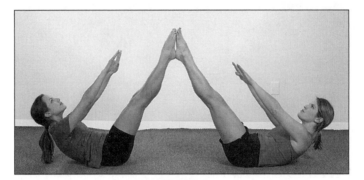

Midpoint.

This cleverly named exercise is a great challenge for the abdominal muscles. Partners anchor their feet together to help stabilize their legs as they move through the exercise. If it is too difficult with legs in the air, partners can perform this exercise with their feet on the ground. Partners should encourage each other not to move their legs while their upper bodies are moving. This will maximize the effort of the abdominal muscles.

Position of Exercisers

Note that both partners exercise at the same time.

◆ Both partners begin by lying supine on the floor, toe-to-toe.

◆ Partners raise their legs off the floor, keeping their feet in contact. This is the same starting position as the partner hundred.

◆ Arms are extended over the head.

Movement

◆ Partners inhale and roll up, lifting their head and shoulders off the ground.

◆ Arms reach out toward toes.

◆ When they get to the top, partners pause and stabilize with the abdominal muscles.

◆ As they exhale, partners roll back down to the starting position, lowering one vertebrae to the floor at a time.

◆ Repeat three to five times.

Back-to-Back Twist

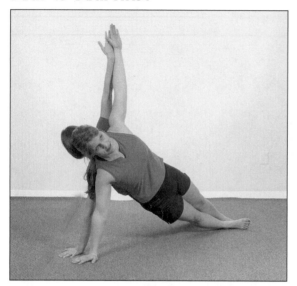

Start/finish.

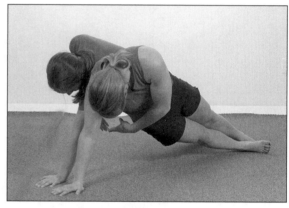

Midpoint.

The twist is a challenging exercise for most new Pilates participants. The twist exercise focuses on rotation at the torso while keeping the abdominals engaged and stabilized. This exercise also improves core stability and muscle control in the upper body. To lessen the intensity, do this exercise with the bottom knee on the ground for support. You can work your way up to the extended leg as you get stronger.

Position of Exercisers

Note that both partners exercise at the same time.

- Partners begin seated back-to-back on the floor, one partner sitting on her right hip and one partner sitting on her left hip, legs extended to the other side.
- The bottom hand is on the floor about one foot away from the hip.

Movement

- Partners push off the bottom foot and hand, extending the legs and straightening the bottom arm.
- The top arm extends straight up to the ceiling.
- Partners rotate their torso, reaching the top hand down and under the bottom arm.
- Partners should encourage each other not to rotate their hips. The rotation should come from the shoulders and torso.
- To maintain spinal stabilization, partners should keep their buttocks and lower back pressed together.
- Return to the starting position.
- Repeat three to five times on each side.

Partner Rolling

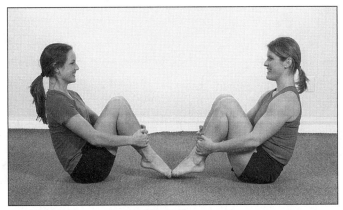

Pose One.

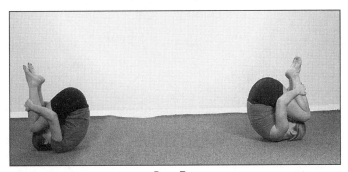

Pose Two.

This exercise allows you to relive your younger days! Rolling like a ball allows for full spinal flexion from the starting position to the finish. Even better, this exercise really massages the back muscles, which can feel great. Partners do this exercise at the same time, facing each other.

Position of Exercisers

Note that both partners exercise at the same time.

◆ Partners begin seated on the floor facing each other.

◆ Pull your knees into your chest, round your back, and tuck your head to your knees and your chin to your chest.

◆ Try to balance with your feet off the floor and your heels pulled in toward your buttocks.

Movement

◆ Inhale, activating the abdominals, and roll back down on to the floor.

◆ Try to roll back all the way to your shoulders, but not all the way back on to your neck.

Partner Swan Dive

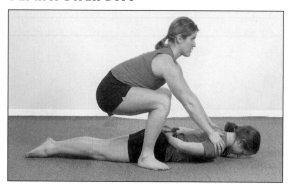

Start/finish.

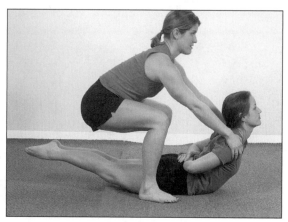

Midpoint.

This exercise encourages extension of the spine. It challenges the core muscles of the abdominals and lower back to extend and lengthen the spine. The spotting partner assists in maximizing the stretch through the shoulders and chest for the exerciser. The spotting partner can also enjoy a stretch through the gluteals by squatting at the end of the stretch.

Position of Exerciser

◆ The exerciser begins by lying prone on the floor with legs extended behind her.

◆ Place your hands on your back, halfway up your spine.

◆ When lying on the floor, lift the pelvis and push the pubic bone into the floor. This will flatten the lumbar portion of the spine.

Position of Spotter

◆ The spotter straddles the exerciser, placing her feet outside of her partner's hips.

◆ Grasp the top of your partner's shoulders and pull gently as she lifts.

Movement

◆ The exerciser lifts her feet toward the spotter's buttocks, making sure her feet and legs stay together and extended.

◆ As she lowers her legs back down to the floor, she scoops her abdominals and, gently pressing her hands into the floor, lifts her chest off the floor.

◆ As she lifts her chest, the spotter assists by pulling gently on the shoulders to heighten the stretch.

◆ As she pulls, the spotter drops her hips toward the stretcher's buttocks and sits in a squatting position.

◆ Repeat six times.

Partner Neck Pull

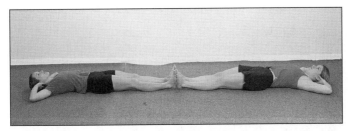

Start/Finish.

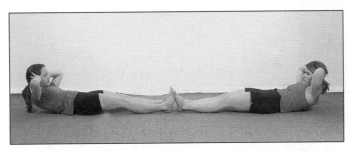

Midpoint.

Sounds like a form of torture, doesn't it? The neck pull is an exercise that stretches the very deep neck muscles that control the movement of the head. When the neck pull is done properly, exercisers can experience a lengthening of the spine from the top of the neck down to the tailbone. However, if either partner has any kind of neck problems, it would be best to skip this exercise.

Position of Exercisers

Note that both partners exercise at the same time.

◆ Both partners begin by lying on the floor facing each other with their legs extended in front of them.

◆ Partners should place the bottoms of their feet against each other's as if they were connected at the feet.

◆ Hands are placed behind the head with the fingertips just below the space where the skull meets the neck. In this position, the fingers can gently lift the head away from the spine.

◆ Elbows are extended wide out to the side and feet are reaching away from the body, pushing against your partner's.

Movement

◆ Partners begin by gently lifting the head and pulling the chin in to the chest, stretching the back of the neck.

◆ As they continue lifting, partners peel the neck and spine off the mat one vertebra at a time.

◆ Partners come up to a seated position and then begin to lower back down to the floor one vertebra at a time.

◆ Repeat six times.

Partner Push-Up

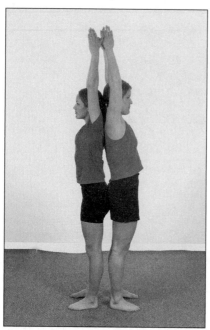

Start/finish.

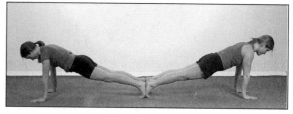

Midpoint.

In addition to the strengthening that comes from executing a traditional push-up in this exercise, exercisers also experience a complete lengthening of the spine during the roll-down portion of the exercise. This action helps to create the space between each vertebra that is so crucial to proper Pilates form. If you cannot do a push-up on your feet, it's okay to do the push-up on your knees in this exercise.

Position of Exercisers

Note that both partners exercise at the same time.

◆ Partners begin by standing back-to-back.

◆ Heels, gluteals, upper backs, and heads are touching in the starting position.

◆ In this standing position, abdominals are engaged and spine should be tall and long.

Movement

◆ Initiating the movement from the top of the head, partners tuck their chins in to their chests and begin a roll-down from the top of the head.

◆ Arms slide down the front of the legs and down to the floor.

◆ When the hands are on the floor, walk them out, lowering the hips to the floor until you are in a push-up position.

◆ Do one push-up.

◆ Walk hands back in toward the body and up the legs.

◆ Roll the spine up one vertebra at a time, bringing your heels, gluteals, upper back, and head back in contact with your partner's.

The Least You Need to Know

- Using a partner for Pilates is an excellent way to introduce this challenging workout routine into your exercise program.

- Pilates is not just for the ultraflexible or fit types. Individuals at all fitness levels can enjoy the benefits that Pilates exercises bring.

- In addition to improving your strength and flexibility, Pilates can help to minimize injuries and improve muscle balance in your body.

- When you have perfected these exercises with your partner, you can try them on your own for a greater challenge.

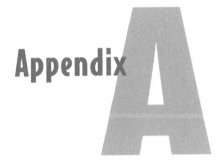

Appendix A

Glossary

adaptation phase The first several weeks of your exercise program when your body is adjusting to the increase in demands.

aerobic activity Aerobic exercise is any activity that uses large muscle groups, is rhythmic, and can be maintained continuously for long periods of time.

body composition The percent of fat versus lean tissue in the body.

chakras Subtle energy centers in the body. The main chakras are situated along the spinal column.

chi In yoga-speak, chi refers to a vital force in the body that is believed to be inherent in all things. The unimpeded circulation of chi and a balance of negative and positive forms in the body are held to be essential to good health in traditional yoga belief.

compound exercises Exercises that involve more than one muscle group. Most often compound exercises involve a group of muscles that act as stabilizers while another group performs the movement.

concentric contraction Refers to the phase of the exercise when the muscle shortens. In most cases, this refers to the flexing part of the movement. During a bicep curl, the concentric contraction occurs when you lift the weight, flexing the elbow.

eccentric contraction Refers to the phase of the exercise when the muscle lengthens. This is usually the extension part of the movement. During a bicep curl, the eccentric contraction occurs when you lower the weight back down, extending the elbow.

endorphins Hormones released into the bloodstream during exercise. These hormones are related to mood elevation, feelings of euphoria, and are the same substances released into the blood stream during sexual arousal.

fascia   The tough connective tissue that surrounds and protects the muscles in the body. It is also responsible for keeping muscle in its proper place in the body.

functional fitness   The body's ability to more easily perform the activities of daily living. It is a new buzzword in the exercise industry. Much exercise training is now geared toward functional fitness instead of simply improving your physical appearance.

muscle function   The specific purpose that the muscle serves during motion.

muscular endurance   The ability of muscles to contract and relax repeatedly over a long period of time against a resistance.

muscular strength   The maximum amount of force muscles are able to exert against a resistance for one repetition.

overload principle   The necessity to push the body beyond its previous limit in order to achieve progress. It's lifting more weight the next day than you did the day before or adding one more city block to your power walk as your fitness improves.

passive stretching   Stretching that is assisted by an outside force.

pedometers   Instruments that measure the distance you travel by foot by responding to the body motion at each step. Pedometers usually clip to a belt or waistband of your pants and track the number of steps you take.

plateau   Any period in development where neither progress nor decline takes place.

posterior lateral rib cage breathing   The description given to the Pilates breath. It involves expanding the posterior lateral rib cage portion of the back on the inhale and letting it fall and collapse on the exhale.

Proprioceptive Neuromuscular Facilitation (PNF)   A stretching technique that involves contracting the muscle and then immediately relaxing it to achieve a deeper stretch.

repetitions   The number of times you will lift the weight per exercise.

Sanskrit   An ancient Indian language from which most yoga terms are derived. It's used mostly for literary and religious purposes today.

set   The number of successive repetitions completed without resting.

spotting   Spotting an exercise means to safely guide the exerciser through the range of motion.

stretch reflex   A neuromuscular action in the body which takes place when a muscle is rapidly stretched. When a muscle is abruptly stretched, the brain sends a signal to that muscle to immediately contract. This prevents the muscle from being overstretched. This is a safety mechanism in the body to help prevent injury.

supersetting   A type of strength-training program that involves completing two different exercises consecutively without rest.

Workout Cards

Workout Log

Name: **Date:**

Notes: **Beginner Strength Workout**

	Exercise	Partner 1 - Set 1	Partner 2 - Set 1	Partner 1 - Set 2	Partner 2 - Set 2	Partner 1 - Set 3	Partner 2 - Set 3
LEGS	Prone Hamstring Curl	—	—	—	—	—	—
	Seated Leg Extension	—	—	—	—	—	—
	MR Leg Lifts	—	—	—	—	—	—
	MR Leg Press	—	—	—	—	—	—
ARMS	MR Bicep Curls	—	—	—	—	—	—
	Hammer Curls	—	—	—	—	—	—
	Dips	—	—	—	—	—	—
	Tricep Extension	—	—	—	—	—	—
CHEST	Standing Chest Press	—	—	—	—	—	—
	Incline Chest Press	—	—	—	—	—	—
	Medicine Ball Pass	—	—	—	—	—	—
BACK	Lat Pull on Ball	—	—	—	—	—	—
	Standing Back Row	—	—	—	—	—	—
	Lying Back Extension	—	—	—	—	—	—
CORE	Partner Sit Up w/Ball	—	—	—	—	—	—
	Tube Twist	—	—	—	—	—	—
	Prone Plank on Knees	—	—	—	—	—	—
SHOULDERS	Lateral Raise w/ Tube	—	—	—	—	—	—
	Shoulder Press	—	—	—	—	—	—
	Front Raise	—	—	—	—	—	—

Workout Log

Name: **Date:**
Notes: Intermediate Strength Workout

	Exercise	Partner 1 - Set 1	Partner 2 - Set 1	Partner 1 - Set 2	Partner 2 - Set 2	Partner 1 - Set 3	Partner 2 - Set 3
LEGS	Partner Squats w/bar	—	—	—	—	—	—
LEGS	Walking Lunges	—	—	—	—	—	—
LEGS	SB Leg Curls	—	—	—	—	—	—
LEGS	SB Adduction	—	—	—	—	—	—
ARMS	Tube Curls on SB	—	—	—	—	—	—
ARMS	Bicep Curls	—	—	—	—	—	—
ARMS	Kneeling Triceps Ext.	—	—	—	—	—	—
ARMS	SB Dips	—	—	—	—	—	—
CHEST	Chest Press Bridge	—	—	—	—	—	—
CHEST	Push Up On SB	—	—	—	—	—	—
CHEST	Chest Press w/Tube	—	—	—	—	—	—
BACK	Lat Pull on SB	—	—	—	—	—	—
BACK	Bent Over Row w/Tube	—	—	—	—	—	—
BACK	Back Extension on SB	—	—	—	—	—	—
CORE	Sidelying Iso Abs	—	—	—	—	—	—
CORE	Incline Crunch on SB	—	—	—	—	—	—
CORE	Medicine Ball Toss	—	—	—	—	—	—
SHOULDER	Sidelying Lateral Raise	—	—	—	—	—	—
SHOULDER	Stork Stance Front Raise	—	—	—	—	—	—
SHOULDER	Shoulder Press on SB	—	—	—	—	—	—

Workout Log

	Exercise	Partner 1 - Set 1	Partner 2 - Set 1	Partner 1 - Set 2	Partner 2 - Set 2	Partner 1 - Set 3	Partner 2 - Set 3
LEGS	Step Ups	—	—	—	—	—	—
	Back to Back Ball Squat	—	—	—	—	—	—
	Lunge w/Transverse Torque	—	—	—	—	—	—
	Single Leg Lunges	—	—	—	—	—	—
ARMS	Stork Stance Arm Curl	—	—	—	—	—	—
	MR Curl with Weights	—	—	—	—	—	—
	SB Triceps Extensions	—	—	—	—	—	—
	Dips on 2 SB	—	—	—	—	—	—
CHEST	SB Chest Fly	—	—	—	—	—	—
	Push up w/MB Roll	—	—	—	—	—	—
	Decline Press Plank	—	—	—	—	—	—
BACK	Stork Stance Lat Pull	—	—	—	—	—	—
	Bent Over Reverse Fly	—	—	—	—	—	—
	Back Extension Ball Toss	—	—	—	—	—	—
CORE	Prone Plank on 2 SB	—	—	—	—	—	—
	Reverse Curl on SB	—	—	—	—	—	—
	MB Partner Toss	—	—	—	—	—	—
SHOULDERS	Rear Delt Row on SB	—	—	—	—	—	—
	Kneeling SB Lat Raise	—	—	—	—	—	—
	Stork Stance Scapulation	—	—	—	—	—	—

Workout Log

Name:
Notes:

Date:

Exercise	Partner 1 - Set 1	Partner 2 - Set 1	Partner 1 - Set 2	Partner 2 - Set 2	Partner 1 - Set 3	Partner 2 - Set 3
LEGS	—	—	—	—	—	—
	—	—	—	—	—	—
	—	—	—	—	—	—
ARMS	—	—	—	—	—	—
	—	—	—	—	—	—
	—	—	—	—	—	—
CHEST	—	—	—	—	—	—
	—	—	—	—	—	—
BACK	—	—	—	—	—	—
	—	—	—	—	—	—
	—	—	—	—	—	—
CORE	—	—	—	—	—	—
	—	—	—	—	—	—
SHOULDERS	—	—	—	—	—	—
	—	—	—	—	—	—

Index

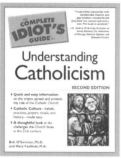
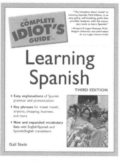
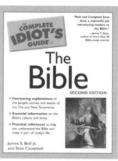
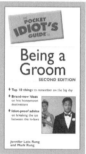
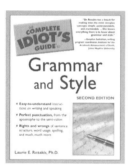
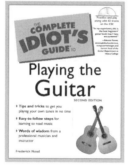
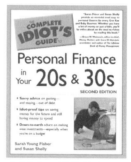
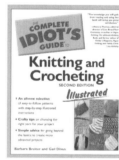
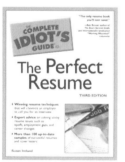
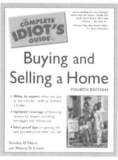
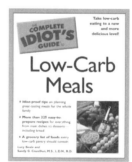
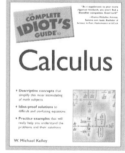